NEW MUSIC 87

Edited by
Michael Finnissy
and Roger Wright

Oxford University Press   1987

Oxford University Press, Walton Street, Oxford OX2 6DP
Oxford New York Toronto
Delhi Bombay Calcutta Madras Karachi
Petaling Jaya Singapore Hong Kong Tokyo
Nairobi Dar es Salaam Cape Town
Melbourne Auckland

and associated companies in
Beirut Berlin Ibadan Nicosia

Oxford is a trade mark of Oxford University Press

Published in the United States
by Oxford University Press, New York

British Library Cataloguing in Publication Data

New music.——1987–
  1. Music
  I. Finnissy, Michael   II. Wright, Roger
  780   ML160
  ISBN 0-19-311928-5
  ISBN 0-19-311926-9 (pbk.)

Typeset by Cotswold Typesetting Ltd., Gloucester
Printed and bound in Great Britain by
Biddles Ltd., Guildford and King's Lynn

CONTENTS

Acknowledgements

Grateful thanks are due to the following for permission to reproduce photographs in this publication: Clive Barda for the scene from Stockhausen's *Donnerstag aus Licht*; Anne Kirchbach for the scene from Young's *Ludwig* in rehearsal; Leslie E. Spatt for the scene from Bintley's *Sons of Horus*; and Zoë Dominic for the scene from Birtwistle's *The Mask of Orpheus*.

The works not acknowledged in the anthology of piano pieces remain in each case the composer's copyright and are reproduced by permission. Every effort has been made to contact owners of copyright material for permission to reproduce copyright music.

Editorial

In the midsummer of 1985 a celebratory event occurred at London's 10 Stratford Place, home of the British Music Information Centre, Electro-Acoustic Music Association, and the Society for the Promotion of New Music. If contemporary music is usually thought of as a Cinderella of the arts today, this was definitely an occasion when she was not moping in front of the fire. Hundreds of people visited the building, enjoyed indoor and outdoor performances, and soaked in a day of new music, unmindful of the so-called 'problem' such music is supposed to present. Perhaps the encouragement we felt at the success of this Open Day sowed the seeds for this journal, hopefully a regular annual celebration, in print, of the varied and various new music happenings in Great Britain.

To cover such a wealth (or simple multiplicity!) of goings-on with equal emphasis to all aesthetic persuasions is, needless to say, impossible. We have, however, tried to cover as much ground as we could, and – in this first issue – give a general, informative picture of the field as well as more detailed coverage of certain areas of it. Consideration is given to two especially vexed areas in the production of music: commissioning (how to offer financial inducements to composers when subtler wiles have proved insufficient) and education (the most obvious outlet for information though neither so welcoming nor unselfish as ideally desirable). Two composer profiles are offered of major figures who continue to lack, at home, the recognition enthusiastically acknowledged elsewhere, and in addition we present contrasting overviews of current and recently past events from home and abroad, listings of various items of interest and importance, and an anthology of short, but thoroughly characteristic piano pieces as perhaps the most tangible representation of compositional activity here.

In this first issue we have concentrated most of the attention on composers, since, after all, they should come first. They are the people who hear the music before any audience does – without them, needless to say, there would not *be* music or concerts – and, although the media and the recording industry underemphasize it (perhaps to pander to what they consider to be popular taste) there are still composers alive today, thousands of them!

One can read many flowery historical accounts of composers' lives – their wranglings with entrepreneurs, performers, and publishers and their constant litany of financial worries, transcending any large-scale socio-economic differences. However, on the whole, composers do not romanticize themselves or needlessly exaggerate their problems, as can be seen in the following articles. It is quite clear that artists are rather badly treated by society. Perhaps nowadays many people can claim such ill-treatment, but the general public expects to be entertained, not to have to entertain, stimulate, or inform, or produce 'art' for the edification or diversion of others. Composers exist, and what they produce stands to represent not only them, but our society too, for the benefit of posterity. In these pages a good many grievances are aired, sometimes with a corollary in suggestions of how things might be improved.

You will, we hope, also find a compositional vitality which is the envy of many countries. Of course, opinions will always differ about whether such vitality is heard in this or that output, but somehow British composers manage these days to remain in the forefront of the world-wide new music scene. Sadly though, there is still a too prevalent notion that a composer's job is something other than writing music; rather, it is to teach, or play the piano, or serve tea at Fortnum and Masons. No! His *job* is to compose music. If we, society at large, place his fundamental self-respect in jeopardy, by devaluing his role in the art-form as a whole, then we, as listeners, performers, entrepreneurs, or anyone even remotely concerned with music, compromise and risk not only the composer's future, but that of music itself as well. Recognition of the discrepancies might serve as an initial corrective.

M.F.
R.W.

BAYAN NORTHCOTT

That was 1985-6 – An Attempted Survey

It was the best of times; it was the worst of times – or just the usual times? How does one, how can one review an entire musical year? Factually? Critically? Trendily? Socio-economically? As a register of individual exploits, or as a play of fads and historical forces? At any rate, chronologically – in so far as one pair of ears could keep up with it all.

What has not lingered in these ears with any vividness is an event which for some was evidently the most important, not just of September 1985, but of the whole season: the British première of Stockhausen's *Donnerstag aus Licht*. Almost exactly 100 years earlier, Bernard Shaw was at critical odds with another vast new import, Gounod's *Mors et Vita*, and there were moments of sweetness and light in Stockhausen's third act when one wondered whether the aim of the two works was that different. The Covent Garden staging was as spectacular as a West End musical, and one had to admire the ambition, not to say nerve, of the Master at his centre-stalls panel, controlling this first instalment of his projected seven-evening saga. But even in the most spiritual, mixed-media-ish structures, there is no substitute for sustained musical thought, and much of the invention of *Donnerstag* struck at least this listener as desultory, anonymous – in fact, as plain poor.

Rather more coherence was to be heard during another September event which may prove to have some future in it: the first Southampton International New Music Week, jointly organized by the University Music Department, Southern Arts, and the Bournemouth Symphony Orchestra, with participation by the Society for the Promotion of New Music. Henze and Goehr were the composers in residence with Oliver Knussen and Simon Bainbridge as supporting composer-conductors. This initial festival failed to solve the problem of attracting a general public, as Huddersfield so remarkably has. But it offered its unconsciously amusing as well as enlightening moments – as when Henze gently attempted to teach the composer of one of the fieriest recent British symphonies, 75 year-old Minna Keal, how to

orchestrate in the manner of Brahms. The most memorable novelty was perhaps Goehr's . . . *a musical offering (J.S.B. 1985)* . . . fresh from its Edinburgh Festival première of the month before. After a decade of relatively sober writing in his new modal figure-bass technique, it seemed Goehr had decided to reintroduce more pungent sounds from his earlier serial period. The resulting sequence of baroque forms simultaneously echoed, parodied, and projected into other historical dimensions by four groups of players certainly provided some of the pawkiest dialectics to be heard from this composer in ages.

Meanwhile the 1985 Proms had brought forth their final commission in the form of Robin Holloway's Viola Concerto: a relatively concise four-movement scheme which effortlessly solved the balance problems of the medium, at least as played by Rivka Golani, but disappointed some ears in its confirmed Elgarian retrogressiveness. In fact Holloway's conscious aspiration in recent years towards (as he hears it) music for use, and music to be loved, has issued in a whole series of modest concerto structures since the *Romanza* for violin and small orchestra of 1976 – others feature oboe, bassoon, harp, and horn – which, performed in sequence, could yet turn out to be more than the sum of their parts: a set of nostalgic English Brandenburgs, almost. Another September première that had, perforce, to aim at more than the sum of its parts was George Benjamin's *Jubilation*, an Inner London Education Authority commission for performance in the Royal Festival Hall not only by the ILEA Schools Symphony Orchestra but by sol-fa-chanting choir, recorder groups, steel bands, and so on from all over the area. Its 10-minute span epitomized Benjamin's gift for striking, well-paced gestures, but stopped just as an enjoyable Ivesian free-for-all seemed in prospect.

Benjamin, Holloway, Goehr, and seventeen other composers all featured in *New Sounds, New Personalities: British Composers of the 1980s*, a book of interviews with Paul Griffiths which appeared from Faber around the beginning of October. As a critic at the centre of the scene, Mr Griffiths could

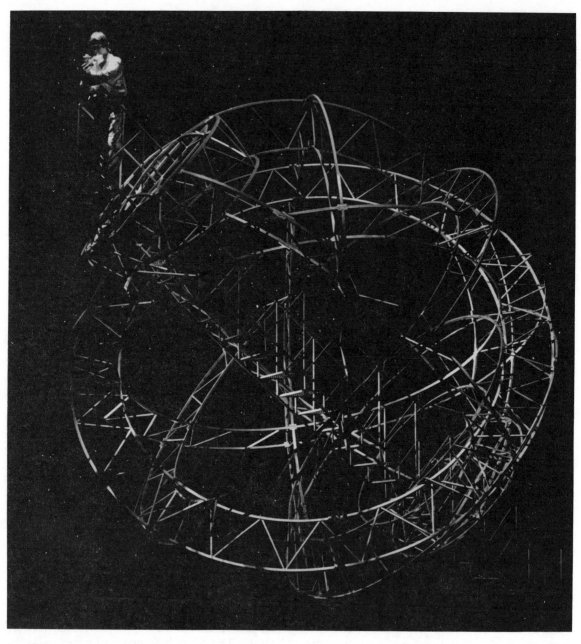

Scene from Karlheinz Stockhausen's *Donnerstag aus Licht*

not perhaps risk the pointed questioning of the Canadian outsider, Murray Schafer, whose *British Composers in Interview* of 1963 provided the acknowledged model. He was also quick to disclaim any intention of setting up a British top 20 – and just as well, since the book did not include Hugh Wood, David Blake, Anthony Payne, or Gordon Crosse, to mention only more established names. None the less the impression of the young and middle-aged ranks of the profession, as it emerged from this cross-section, was of an encouraging culture and diversity – except doubtless to the kind of disgruntled practitioner who writes periodically to *The Listener* complaining that the whole show is run by a serialist-avant-garde mafia.

The most imposing October event ought to have been IRCAM in London: three concerts of electro-acoustic music commissioned by that institute and presented in St John's, Smith Square by Radio 3, with Boulez himself to expatiate upon the wonderful possibilities of his new 'real time' 4X computer. In fact, the British première of *Alba*, four Beckett settings for mezzo-soprano and ensemble by our own Nigel Osborne, proved relatively cautious in deploying its computer-generated tape essentially as a tutti-amplifying device. Some of the French works showed no such restraint and amid the welter of voices, instruments, tape, and 'real time' electronics of Philippe Manoury's *Zeitlauf*, one recalled all the more feelingly Stravinsky's belief that, 'My freedom will be so much the greater and more meaningful the more narrowly I limit my field of action.' Not that Colin Matthews exactly seemed to have recalled it in the month's most spectacular first performance. Rarely can even the London Sinfonietta under Oliver Knussen have faced such a virtuoso challenge as *Suns Dance*, commissioned for the opening of the third (and presumably last) series of Music of Eight Decades. Yet the perpetual thematic evolution of this 17-minute rampage – there is virtually no repeated material – must have demanded its own compositional discipline; certainly the piece emerged as strikingly different from Matthews's more darkly romantic scores of recent years.

November began badly with the death of Hans Keller – for 40 years arch-enemy of all phonies, incompetents, and drears, mentor of many of the finest composers and performers, and irreplaceable medium of musicality at its deepest. At least it was soon clear that his legacy of writings, including three unpublished books and unnumbered essays, analyses, polemics, and letters for the anthologizing, was sufficient to influence our musical life for years to come. Whether he would have approved of many of the items in the four-concert series of British and international novelties given by the tireless Arditti String Quartet in the Almeida Theatre might be doubted – almost certainly not of the electronic string instruments by Raad of Canada which the Arditti introduced in their first concert, though the incessant collective scraping of Michael Nyman's minimalist new Quartet (1985), commissioned as a demonstration piece, made their individual qualities difficult to judge. Of other November premières, Brian Elias's *Geranos*, commissioned by the Fires of London, impressed with its sustained balance between a grittily atavistic rhetoric and a sensuousness of almost Ravelian delicacy, while Maxwell Davies's school cantata, *First Ferry to Hoy*, adapted sounds from his recent symphonies

to *Noye's Fludde*-type forces to evoke a vision of a school of whales – its Queen Elizabeth Hall impact reinforced by a passionate plea for more spending on music in state schools from the composer himself.

Most widely noticed, however, was the SPNM Orchestral Composition Award Concert given by the Royal Liverpool Philharmonic under Nicholas Cleobury in the Philharmonic Hall and at the Barbican with generous funds from the Ralph Vaughan Williams Trust. It was a pity that one of the chosen scores – Glyn Perrin's *Tu, même* – proved too difficult to rehearse in the time. Of the others, Michael Rosenzweig's brooding *Symphony in One Movement* was more memorable for its complex textural ebb and flow than for its basic ideas, but its composer's musicality was never in doubt. Steve Martland's *Babi Yar* turned out to be a longer, louder cut off the same roll of aggressive Dutch-style systems music as his *American Invention* and horn concerto, *Orc*, heard earlier in the year. The composer claimed it as a 'confrontation' of the historical atrocity of the title, though it was difficult to see how that could be. A few days later, under the rubric of Response and with the connivance of the GLC, the London Sinfonietta tried a more sybaritic way with new music by offering a whole weekend of free concerts and related events in the Royal Festival Hall 'Music Box' for anyone prepared to wander in with a drink and to plump themselves down on a scatter cushion. Once there they admittedly had to put up with torrid heating, horrid acoustics, and the periodic rumbling of Hungerford railway bridge. All the same, thanks to such artists as Oliver Knussen and the players themselves, a pleasant atmosphere emerged. Among many recent pieces (more or less) heard were *The Shorelines of Certainty*, a delicate study in rocking ostinati by Jonathan Lloyd, and a reworking by Mark-Anthony Turnage of his nervy jazz nocturne, *Before Dark*, under the more insinuating title of *After Dark*.

Berio's 50th birthday was the focus of the Huddersfield Contemporary Music Festival in November, culminating in a reading by BBC forces of his *Coro* which many felt revealed the work's full stature for the first time. And Berio celebrations continued in London during December – notably a warmly received London Sinfonietta concert including the British première of *Requies*. But it was David Matthews who bore the brunt of the month's critical scrutiny with two major orchestral novelties: his half-hour tone-poem, *In the Dark Time*, given by the BBC SO under Mark Elder in

London, and his Third Symphony launched by the Hallé Orchestra under Bryden Thomson in Manchester. Of these, the more recent and often lustrously scored evocation of the passing of winter proved the less cohesive in overall form; the tightly-worked one-movement Symphony drew some fire for its almost polemical conservatism of idiom, but its slow epilogue with solo oboe rhapsodizing away while the strings serenely teased out the work's tonal tensions certainly continued to haunt this hearer. Meanwhile, the sadly early death of the composer and translator, Bill Hopkins, was commemorated in a New Macnaghten concert by Jane Manning and Music Projects/London under Richard Bernas. Pupil of Messiaen and Barraqué, Hopkins may have aspired to the glittering anonymity of French avant-garderie of the 1950s, currently so out of fashion. But of his few completed works, the fine-spun word setting and pointillistic scoring of *Sensation* (1965), on texts of Rimbaud and Beckett, sounded quite as convincing as his models.

Robert Ponsonby bowed out at the year's turning after 13 seasons as BBC Controller, Music, having, it was generally felt, sustained the progressive policies of his predecessor, Sir William Glock, firmly backed his own choices such as Rozhdestvensky and Sir John Pritchard, and survived with dignity such traumas as the 1980 Musicians' Union strike and Robert Simpson's pamphlet, *The Proms and Natural Justice*. Since he had already planned the 1986 Proms, the policies of his successor could hardly emerge until the autumn of that year; it was noted that John Drummond had subsumed both Radio and Television responsibilities but it was not clear whether his acceptance of an initial contract for three years only was by preference or because Dr Simpson's arguments had hit home after all.

Of January's new offerings, the Opera Factory London Sinfonietta première of *Hell's Angels* – words by its producer, David Freeman, music by Nigel Osborne – was so generally panned that a subsequent newsletter from its publisher even went so far as to hint at possible collusion among the London critics (some hope!). In fact this ironic pointing of a parallel between the divine retribution of syphilis in the fifteenth century and the latter-day arrival of AIDS had its clever one-liners and some serely suggestive music, but its combination of less than coherent tendentiousness with paralytic pacing proved fatal. Less varied than anticipated, too, was the SPNM's major public concert of the season by the National Centre for

Orchestral Studies SO under Adrian Leaper, in that all four of the chosen works were concerned with images of darkness and disquiet. The smoothly skilled techniques of at least two of them – Martin Butler's post-Bax tone-poem, *The Flights of Col*, and Silvina Milstein's more Schoenbergian *Sombras* – also suggested the dangers of composers working in too academic a milieu, and only John Woolrich's slow processional, *A Song of the Dark*, with its elegiac chorus of low flutes, left a personal sound in the memory. But the month's most striking first performance was surely Nicholas Sackman's *Corranach* by Lontano under Odaline de la Martinez: a sustained variation structure, now remote, now raucous, inspired by a droll description of a Scottish funeral out of Smollett and not only revealing an unsuspected dead-pan humour but confirming Sackman as one of the strongest long-term prospects of his generation.

Edmund Rubbra slipped quietly away in February aged 84 – a neglected figure except on Lyrita records and, periodically, Radio 3, less perhaps for the conservatism of his idiom than for the sheer uneven vastness of his output. But it was hard to believe that the individual plangency of his best music – for instance, his Second String Quartet, G minor Piano Concerto, or Fourth, Sixth, and Seventh Symphonies – would be forgotten for good; nor his broadminded solicitude in the memory of his many students. And suddenly with his passing, together with the inactivity of Sir Lennox Berkeley, the fact that Alan Bush had just celebrated his 85th birthday and that even the eternal Tippett was now an unlikely octogenarian, one became aware of a strange gap in the English succession: that the deaths of Lutyens, Searle, and Britten and the longstanding US residencies of Fricker and Hamilton leaves the intensely independent Simpson as virtually our only substantial composer in the sixties-seventies age-group – and he has recently retreated to Ireland. It seems that with the Goehr-Birtwistle-Maxwell Davies generation only just into its fifties we may in time have to adjust to some very youthful Grand Old Men.

A new Violin Sonata from Simpson was one of February's novelties: chunky and hard-driven in its outer movements, as projected by Pauline Lowbury with Christopher Green-Armytage, but including some of his subtlest fugal writing. A few days later the London Sinfonietta under Diego Masson brought forth Mark-Anthony Turnage's *On All Fours*, obliquely based upon baroque forms but actually another of his punchy modern jazz concertantes with much sultry work for John

Harle's saxophone. Space was also made for George Benjamin to play three of his recent piano pieces, including the lolloping new *Fantasy on Iambic Rhythm*, which, together with *Jubilation*, comprised the bulk of his completed work for over three years. The flair and ebullience of the writing, not to say the playing, were memorable; less so, the melodic and contrapuntal substance. There was counterpoint to excess in James Erber's new *Music for 25 solo strings*, premièred by Odaline de la Martinez's Contemporary Chamber Orchestra, yet this progressive overlaying of a chord sequence derived from a Byrd motet retained a Tippett-like incandescence for all Erber's studies with Ferneyhough. The closely-woven atonal tissue of Bernard Benoliel's variations-cum-Yeats-setting, *The Dark Tower*, revived in the same concert, made a less immediately personal impression, though this is an earlier work of a composer whose small but blackly visionary output – notably his majestic, once-broadcast Symphony – has yet to be generally recognized for its true, if unsettling, worth.

March began with another act of restitution in a remarkably proficient new production by the Guildhall School of Music and Drama of Nicholas Maw's opera, *The Rising of the Moon*, totally neglected in this country since its original Glyndebourne runs of 1970–1 – either because its romantic comedy genre was deemed too 'culinary' or its story of the British Army worsted in nineteenth-century Ireland too politically 'sensitive' – yet coming up, a few patches of overly busy music apart, as a richly effective, not to say funny piece, full of harmony and invention. At the opposite extreme came the British première in concert form of three massive tableaux from Messiaen's *Saint François d'Assise* by Fischer-Dieskau and BBC forces under Seiji Ozawa in the presence of the composer, in which a fervour and vividness of sonorous imagery mostly triumphed over a by-now pretty shortwinded norm of formal articulation – though it was a shame that the tableau with the birds was not included, in which Messiaen's abandonment for once of his beloved piano had resulted in some of his most novel textures in recent years.

Among the month's concert premières, Robert Saxton's one-movement chamber symphony, *The Circles of Light*, launched by the London Sinfonietta under Esa-Pekka Salonen, was received with exceptional warmth: the latest in a series of spiritually inspired pieces exploiting a kind of spiral form in which various circulating textures tend towards a moment of transcendence, it also proved

the hardest, brightest, most fiercely sustained of them. Yet its fierceness was as nothing compared with the 40-minute turmoil of Birtwistle's major new orchestral piece, *Earth Dances*, an awesome monumentalization of his recent interest in generating structure from the interplay of simultaneous, registrally distinct and often hyperactive 'strata'. In the event, the no-holds-barred reading by the BBC SO under Peter Eötvös drew mixed reactions, from the critic who hailed it as 'a *Rite of Spring* for our time' to those who wondered whether Birtwistle's evident broadening of style had not admitted an element of corny gesture, or who felt that the incessant stratification precluded silence as a punctuating device. But Birtwistle had at least included one bar of stasis near the end, expressly in memory of the critic, Brigitte Schiffer, who had died in January: a touching moment for those long familiar with her crop-haired, kindly-acerbic ubiquity at contemporary events and her distinctively Continental angle on the English scene.

Towards the end of March, the expiring GLC had funded the London Sinfonietta in another Response weekend, highlighting the music of Kurtag; at the beginning of April, the public suddenly found itself faced with the new South Bank Board which, in recognition of the eight and three-quarter million pounds the Government had grudgingly divulged for its first year of operations at least, had graciously consented not to resign even before coming into existence after all. 'Don't expect anything to happen for ages,' its Chairman Ronald Grierson told the press with reference to the inherited events and whatnot yet to be worked through. Still, the General Director (Arts), Nicholas Snowman, fresh from IRCAM, was soon warming to his plans for converting the QEH to take small-scale opera and for coaxing more 'thematic' planning from the four London orchestras with a 'Beethoven plus' series here, a 'Brahms-Schoenberg' package there, perhaps a festival of 'late' works to go with Sir Peter Hall's proposed cycle of late Shakespeare at the National Theatre, and so on. The autumn of 1988 was to see the first collaboration of all the South Bank institutions in a new contemporary arts festival entitled 'Perspectives '88', which would spotlight Messiaen at 80, Lutoslawski, Steve Reich, *et al*. At this point someone was heard to murmur that these estimable figures already did quite well in Britain, thank you (Reich, for instance, had only recently completed an Arts Council Contemporary Music Network tour). But Mr Snowman was quick to refer to his proposed New Music Review in which novelties from foreign festivals would be zipped straight over to the Metropolis – 'and from Huddersfield, too,' he added when the obvious question about the native product seemed to threaten. It was all very hopeful. And, as they say, we shall see.

The world's leading creative figures continued to descend on London, in any case. April brought both Carter and Lutoslawski; the one tearing himself away from his Fourth String Quartet in progress to hear the Arditti give the first three in readings of tremendous dash, if a little lightweight in expression, and the other to direct the British première of his violin concerto *Chain 2*, quite a lengthy piece, immaculate as ever, if by now stretching the familiar devices pretty thin. Meanwhile Gordon Crosse re-emerged after a somewhat reclusive year or so with a substantial Piano Trio for the young Hartley Trio in the Wigmore Hall, in which the second of its two movements battered away with a Beethovenian dynamism quite new in his music. Robin Holloway's half-hour tone-poem *Seascape and Harvest*, commissioned for the City of Birmingham Symphony Orchestra, was more a matter of these you have loved – the 'you' in this case being the work's dedicatee, Simon Rattle. Indeed, so manifold and rhapsodic were the allusions to Wagner, Mahler, Strauss, Elgar, Ravel, even Gershwin, that the introduction and allegro structure arguably failed to establish a central momentum. But many of its quieter passages were radiantly realized and its Birmingham Town Hall première certainly came over *con amore*.

It was around this time that Londoners began to suffer from a strange surfeit of single-composer festivals. At the beginning of March there had been an intensive four-day Penderecki festival at the Royal Academy of Music with the great man himself, shortly followed by a Rodrigo festival similarly graced on the South Bank. A projected Ginastera festival in early April had failed to find adequate funds, but the elegant participation of Richard Rodney Bennett in a whole variety of events celebrating his 50th birthday almost amounted to a festival in itself. And now, at the beginning of May, for no very obvious reason, the London Symphony Orchestra suddenly laid on a lavish Bernstein festival at the Barbican with the maestro, 67 years not withstanding, leaping to the podium to claim due adulation and conducting two of the concerts. Of British contemporaries, only Britten was included as comrade-in-arms, though early Knussen might have been chosen to illustrate the influence. As for all that Bernstein itself – from the severities of the *Jeremiah Symphony*

to the razmatazz of *Mass* (another superb Guildhall School effort) – one suddenly had the curious feeling that the reason why, for all its ebullience, none of it sounded quite fresh, was not its surface eclecticism but its underlying compositional technique – of all things, its academicism.

Absolutely nothing of the academy about Birtwistle's 'source opera', *The Mask of Orpheus*, which finally achieved its première at the London Coliseum later in the month – but then no contemporary composer has remade himself a technique more single-mindedly out of an idiosyncratic view of the sonic raw materials of music and of time itself. If the vast three-act structure none the less came over as more the rounding-off of a phase than the inception of a new one, this was doubtless partly due to the near decade-long delay in its completion and staging, during which the public has also had quite a dose of slow, ritualistic music-theatre pieces from Messiaen, Stockhausen, Glass, and company. Certainly the keening lyricism and grinding chorale textures of the first two acts belonged to the early 1970s world of *The Triumph of Time*, and while the third act, added in 1983, proved more volatile in its textural cross-cutting, it came over as a pendant to the main dramatic action rather than its culmination – at least in the somewhat shortened form presented. Whether or not the skill with which the producer and designer, David Freeman and Jocelyn Herbert, had clarified Peter Zinovieff's labyrinthine libretto also undercut the work's potential grandeur, its musical presentation, under the direction of Elgar Howarth, was generally accounted a triumph for the forces of English National Opera, while Birtwistle's extensive tape interpolations were found especially striking. In fact the opera became something of a cult during its run, with enthusiasts seeing it several times.

June's most publicized première was of Maxwell Davies's Violin Concerto, given by Isaac Stern and the Royal Philharmonic under André Previn as the highlight of the tenth St Magnus Festival and broadcast live on TV and Radio from Orkney to the world, with a London première four days later. It proved somewhat bemusing, for while its pitch procedures seemed as arcane as ever, its structure edged even closer to nineteenth-century models than before: a cyclic three-movement form complete with distant Pibroch, almost like a latter day Max Bruch. But its relative concision and clarity of orchestration suggested an advance on the earlier symphonies and there were beautiful moments. Divergent aspects of Maw were also to be heard in a brace of novelties around the beginning of the month. The *Sonata Notturna* for cello and strings, held over from the 1985 King's Lynne Festival and launched in the town's Fermoy Centre by the passionate Alexander Baillie and the Peterborough String Orchestra, harked elegantly back to the crepuscular scurryings of the earlier *Life Studies* and *Sinfonia*. By contrast, *Personae IV–VI* for solo piano at the Bath Festival resumed the more exploratory manner (if not quite the opaque harmony) of the first three *Personae* of 1973 in formidable sweeps of invention challenging Peter Donohoe's virtuosity to the utmost. Maw's admirers were delighted to learn that he had now embarked on the final haul of his vast orchestral *Odyssey*, fitfully in progress for over a decade, for definite first performance at the 1987 Proms.

Of the high summer festivals, the Almeida burst at the seams as ever with offerings rich and strange – from Music of the New Spain to Steve Reich at 50, from wall to wall Takemitsu to à la recherche du Arvo Pärt – though it was Oliver Knussen's short *Frammenti da Chiara*, serenely delivered by the ladies of the BBC Chorus under Simon Joly, that hovered in the mind. A slow, canonic litany – modern Palestrina, almost – rather different from Knussen's usual more mosaic continuities, this proved to be a layer of a processional 'something to do with St Clare, something to do with angels,' which he planned to complete for the Proms with additional sections and orchestral layerings – though in the event he failed to. Meantime, the Cheltenham Festival had brought forth Robert Saxton's Viola Concerto with the Scottish Chamber Orchestra accompanying the dynamic young Paul Silverthorne: a work closer to traditional dialectics than *The Circles of Light*, but exploiting a comparable mode of textural rustlings and *frissons*, it did just raise the question as to whether the continuities of these undeniably fluent and effective pieces rested upon rather too even and incessant a revolving of the total chromatic.

But July most notably brought to a head the 60th birthday celebrations of that by now almost honorary Englishman (or Cat?) Hans Werner Henze. These had begun months before with a whole sequence of the chamber works spread through the Nash Ensemble's Austro-German winter series at the Wigmore Hall. In March, the London Sinfonietta had mounted a semi-staged performance of *Elegy for Young Lovers* in the QEH – that ambiguous confection of arty libretto and delectable sounds – and a whole sequence of the operas had been offered on Radio 3 in the early summer. At the Brighton Festival in May, Peter

Donohoe had marvellously pulled together the sprawling Second Piano Concerto. In June, Henze had been composer-in-residence at the Aldeburgh Festival and in evidence at the Almeida, and now came the British première of his huge four-movement Seventh Symphony at the Proms: a dedicated reading by the CBSO under Simon Rattle in which, as the composer exclaimed in evident astonishment, one could actually hear every note. The question was indeed whether half those teeming notes were necessary; whether there was not an even greater disparity than ever between nondescript material and wastefully elaborate textures. On the other hand, the way Henze had blocked out the work as a series of vast crescendos, articulated in well-timed switches between contrasting colouristic paragraphs certainly suggested a new firmness of aim – not to speak of wowing the Promenaders.

The two actual 1986 Proms commissions proved a little disappointing. Gordon Crosse's *Array* for trumpet and strings, featuring the stentorian young Norwegian soloist, Håkan Hardenberger, was apparently an attempt to develop the kind of bright, simple material for which he has always shown a gift in a form of diatonic serialism, but – whether owing to the demands of some undivulged programme or whatever – it ran on into diffuseness. In his *Madonna of Winter and Spring*, Jonathan Harvey brought the BBC SO under Peter Eötvös and an array of synthesizers, ring modulators, and loudspeakers – not to say his, by now, considerable expertise in mixing such resources – to bear on a simple 'redemptive' programme suggested by its section headings: Conflict, Descent, Depths, Mary. To object that the work's 40-minute progress, while often ravishing in sound, seemed perilously simplistic in substance was doubtless to miss Harvey's meditative point. But if meditation was the aim, one could not help questioning the point of all that troublesome technology when any drone, repeat pattern, or mantra would do as well.

The rival show down at the South Bank, retitled 'Summerscope' and directed by the London Sinfonietta's Michael Vyner, at least had the year's third major novelty from Birtwistle to flaunt – and in a QEH in which the South Bank Board had duly fulfilled its first promise of installing an operatic stage (to the vast clarification of the acoustics, incidentally). This was the 90-minute television commission, *Yan Tan Tethera*, an allegory of rival shepherds from North and South and their choruses of sheep, of which David Freeman's Opera Factory production could be criticized only for underplaying the more formalistic aspects of this 'mechanical pastoral', as Birtwistle has called it. A few lines of Tony Harrison's text and the folksy, vibratoless delivery required of Omar Ebrahim's Northern shepherd perhaps strayed across the tenuous divide between the primitivistic and the *faux-naif*, but the tapestry of sounds woven by the small accompanying ensemble from behind a gauze was a continuous, luminous fascination. Summerscope also brought forth a concentrated concert commission in Dominic Muldowney's Sinfonietta, given by the London Sinfonietta under Diego Masson: a four-movements-in-one attempt to see if the classical tonic–dominant tension could be reactivated as a formal force – though, Muldowney being the foxiest of our younger composers, the experiment was conducted with such teasing obliqueness that it would take several hearings to determine whether he had pulled it off.

Nor was the Edinburgh Festival, despite its recent dramatic leanings, without one commission. Having been handed a whole weekend of concerts to programme to his taste, Goehr had invoked *You, Always You*, a 10-minute ensemble piece, from his one-time pupil, Geoffrey King, who might by now be quite established had he made London instead of Edinburgh his centre of operations. As projected by Lontano under Odaline de la Martinez, this interplay of polymetrical lines achieved a real, cumulative ardour without ever lapsing into the dreaded 'New Romanticism'. Two other provincial premières belatedly caught up with ought to come in here: Robert Simpson's Eleventh String Quartet, of which the first performance by the Coull Quartet reached Radio 3 in August, proved in its continuous four-movement trajectory one of the most tightly structured and variously characterized of the series, while Colin Matthews's two-movement Second Quartet, heard in a tape of its Endellion Quartet tour, turned out in its mostly muted progress his most intricately sensitized nightmusic to date.

At which point this chronicler is overcome with remorse at what he missed: ensembles such as the Northern Sinfonia doing their bit for new music with concerto commissions from Holloway and Edward Cowie; invaluable *second* performances from the Royal Liverpool Philharmonic sponsored by the Melos Trust of Harvey's *Whom Ye*

Adore and Geoffrey Poole's *Visions*: the Aldeburgh Festival commission, *Le Livre de Fauvel*, which, according to all who heard it, marked the impressive arrival of its composer, Rupert Bawden. And not just out of London, either: what of the remarkable variety of events mounted by the Electro-Acoustic Music Association of Great Britain over the year, or the Endymion Ensemble's valuable retrospectives of Knussen, Bainbridge, Osborne, and Muldowney, or the stream of 'unofficial' concerts at the British Music Information Centre (whose innovatory young director of eight years, Roger Wright, was lost to the BBC at the end of the present period)? And what indeed of James Dillon's sizeable London Sinfonietta commission of June, *Uberschreiten*, which this writer did hear, but has forgotten to include in its proper place – perhaps because its 23-minute span of textural waves and freezings onto a refrain chord, though exceptionally clear in scoring compared with some of the products of the 'New Complexity', seemed to remain on the level of mere *montage sonore?*

Yet a compositional scene ranging all the way from the 'New Complexity' to the 'New Romanticism' that offered its composers, especially the young, such a range of opportunities, and to which those young generally responded with so high a level of skill, was surely to be accounted basically healthy – except possibly on the Boulezian grounds that its very plurality represented a betrayal of historical purpose. Or was it? Considering the financial policies of a philistine Government, it was heartening how surprisingly few new musical enterprises actually folded during the year. But the truncation of Adrian Jack's eccentrically adventurous 1986 MusICA series at the ICA was an ominous portent and by mid-summer the opera companies, including ENO, had announced plans of drastic retrenchment inimical to risky new work. Moreover, the dilemma of a musical community increasingly beholden to commercial patronage is not only a direct one of sometimes having to compromise programme choices. There was an increasingly insidious effect in a more-than-ever competitive Press, where music critics – with the exception of a few publications – found themselves under pressure to tackle trendy 'issues' and to churn out preview material, profiles, and chat; the kind of material which,

however well intentioned and at whatever remove, must inevitably advance the interests of the sponsors, the agents, and the record companies. Never did it seem more urgent to press the argument that for the vitality of music, or for any of the arts, there can be no substitute for informed, individual, independent after-the-event *criticism*.

Even the reprieve of serious music broadcasting from the influence of advertising proposed by the Peacock Report could only be taken as temporary given that the licence system would be bound to re-emerge as a political issue in due course and the longer-term proliferation of commercial media likely to undermine a national, public-service broadcasting ideal. This is an eventuality all musicians ought to fear, for, whatever sins of bias or omission might be laid at the doors of the BBC Music Division, its very existence as musical employer and patron and the fact that a first performance relayed from London is instantaneously available to interested listeners in the farthest corners of the realm, has for 60 years remained overwhelmingly the single most cohesive and beneficent factor in our musical life.

Yet the underlying anxiety as far as new music was concerned remained as ever – who needs it? Not, apparently, the bulk of the general public, unless educationally caught young. Nor was much left of the old social functions whereby even the greatest composers had to grind out contredanses for the Redoutensaal, Albumblätter for the parlour piano trade, or Verismo for the opera circuit; 'serious' and 'popular' were more divided worlds than ever and most 'applied' music, from films to factory farms, was now the work of specialists or machines. Great music ultimately creates its own need, and doubtless it was such a principle of hope that kept composers, from the venerable Tippett to the sprightly young Judith Weir, at work on major projects throughout the period under review. But was that substitute for older modes of patronage, the commissioning system as it has burgeoned since the last war, anything more than an artificial stimulus? And did it tend to place a premium on striking mannerism rather than substantial musical thought? And why did there nevertheless seem to be ever more aspiring composers? These were just some of the questions that found no ready answer in 1985–6.

ROGER WRIGHT

Commissioning – The Debate Continues

Over the past two years I have been involved in discussions about how composers are commissioned. These have taken place between the Arts Council, the Regional Arts Associations, composers, and their representative bodies – the Composers' Guild and the Association of Professional Composers. I was asked to take part in the debates because I 'wore three hats' and was, therefore, apparently, 'acceptable' to all sides. My work at the British Music Information Centre in the promotion of British music caused me to be seen as an impartial supporter of all our composers. As I also served on music advisory panels of both the Arts Council and the Greater London Arts Association (London's regional arts association), I was regarded as sitting on both sides of the devolution debate fence. This so-called 'devolution debate' stems from the Arts Council's infamous report *The Glory of the Garden*. On the devolution issue, perhaps the most significant paragraph of the report is the following:

> The Council will also be considering, in consultation with the Regional Arts Associations, the transfer to them of responsibility for as many of the Council's current block allocations (providing for one-off grants for particular purposes under a variety of general schemes) as can be equally well handled by the Associations.

This paragraph set the scene for the battle – and it *is* a battle – over commissioning between the Arts Council and the Regional Arts Associations (RAAs). One might have thought that these two groups would work together on this and all other issues but instead there has been much disagreement about the role of the RAAs in relation to the central Arts Council in general and constant argument about who should fund this or that commission in particular.

As an impartial outsider I was called upon to take part in, and often chair, various meetings concerning commissions and found myself caught in the cross-fire between the Council and RAAs. From the battleground emerged a series of mud-dled policies which are still under discussion. This autobiographical introduction therefore merely serves to explain the resulting impossibility of writing the article about commissioning I had originally intended.

This section of the yearbook had the working title 'Commissioning: how to do it, how much it costs, and who pays for it.' This might seem to be an easy task to undertake. All it should require is a few paragraphs about why commissioning new work is so vital, then an advisory section on how to select a composer, a scale of recommended fees, and a list of the funding bodies. Life would be simple then for would-be commissioners. Once fired with enthusiasm to commission, they would select a composer, arrange a deadline for delivery of the music, check to see what he or she should be paid, and approach the necessary funding body for financial assistance, if the commissioner is unable to fund the necessary amount themselves. Alas, this article cannot be so straightforward because the business of commissioning has become a bureaucratic minefield and political football. Ultimately of course, it is the composers and their music – ironically the existence of which is the chief reason for commissioning – who suffer most as a result of this lack of clear guide-lines. I still believe wholeheartedly in the commissioning of new work – it is, after all, the life blood of our musical world – but this article can be nothing more than a cautionary tale rather than a series of helpful guide-lines on the dos and don'ts.

I might have been regarded as a useful arbitrator to the arts funding organizations, but there is one aspect of this commissioning debate about which I am certainly not impartial; namely that we should rejoice in composers' burning desire to write music and also acknowledge his or her difficulty in doing so without the necessary funding. The tiresome old argument about composers working best in adverse conditions should not have a place at the end of the twentieth century. If a composer cannot afford to pay the rent how can he afford to think and write. In Professor Alan Rump's excellent report for the Arts

Council entitled *How We Treat our Composers*, Hugo Cole is quoted as follows:

> In status, the composer heads his profession. Every musician who has committed notes to paper would prefer to be thought of as a composer . . . Yet composers as a class are not particularly contented people. They have resigned themselves to living thriftily, while others with half their talent grow affluent. But almost all want the approval of the society they live in; approval which seems to be withheld when society does not even grant them a living wage. The peculiar view of life which lies at the root of their being and accounts for their creative ability – the intransigence that leads them to insist on the validity of their personal vision, and to demand that things should go their and no other way – unfits them for accepting the judgements of others or fitting comfortably into the social scheme of things. Most have, if not a grudge against society, a certain sadness at heart, because their works – which are their children – are too little noticed, praised, and understood. . . . Society venerates composers, but can get along without them; pats them on the head, then tells them to run away and play.[1]

As Professor Rump himself pointed out elsewhere in his report, it is too easy to be complacent about the predicament in which composers find themselves today. Of course composition flourishes now more abundantly in Britain than it did earlier in this century. The opportunities to be given commission fees, first performances, and broadcasts have multiplied considerably. However, as Rump states,

> the new opportunities are having to be shared out amongst a profession that has swollen since the mid-sixties with the expansion of higher music education and the place of composition within it.[2]

In other words we are faced with a situation in which we have more composers in Britain than ever before and, instead of using them to good advantage we are finding it difficult to support them adequately. The funding for the arts, (and the new arts in particular), is increasingly under threat and so only a tiny percentage of our composers is receiving funding for new work.

This would seem to be the ideal opportunity for the Arts Council to step into the arena and present a coherent overview of composers' problems with some strong guide-lines and policies. There is, of course, no instant solution to the problem of 'too many composers, too little money' but there are basic questions regarding the funding of composers in general and commissioning in particular which remain untackled, let alone unresolved.

In the Arts Council's defence, it has to be stated that, since the Rump report, it has accepted the need for an increase in commission fee levels. In 1985–6 the Council considered applications for commission funding in the light of guide-line figures which allowed for a 15 to 20 per cent increase in fees. The Council believed that it was making a contribution towards an increase in the fees paid to composers, which had generally been considered to be too low. However, although some RAAs have accepted these new guide-line levels, other RAAs felt that they were too high. There is therefore no general agreement throughout the country concerning guide-lines for fees in commissioning.

In addition to this confusion over fee levels, there is similar uncertainty in other aspects of commissioning. It is true that, although limited progress has been made on the uniformity of fee levels, procedures have become more standardized in recent years. However, there are still some wide variations in the approaches to commission applications taken by RAAs and ourselves. Perhaps the most glaring examples of inconsistency are those connected with part-funding of commissions. Several RAAs may make the provision of outside funding a condition of any support given.

The procedures referred to below are the areas of commissioning policy which differ from region to region:

a) that the option of part-funding with another funding organization should be considered;
b) that 'incestuous' applications for commission funding should not be considered – i.e. ensembles should not consider commissioning members of the ensemble;
c) that applications should not be considered from student composers;
d) that applications should not be considered for commissions awarded retrospectively;
e) that commissioned works should have the prospect of several scheduled performances after the first;
f) that the awarding of copying costs should be discretionary.

---

1 Alan Rump, *How we Treat our Composers*, Arts Council Publication, p. 255.
2 Ibid., p. 256.

It must also be remembered that, in addition to these regional differences, there is further confusion provided by the decision that some commission applications will continue to be considered by the central Arts Council. They are as follows:

a) where the value of the commission according to the fee guide-lines is in excess of £4,000;
b) where the first performance of the work is not scheduled within a Regional Arts Association area;
c) where work is commissioned for the Contemporary Music Network.

The devolution of money to the regions for commissioning has confused the application procedure for commission money. In the past, commissioners applied to the Arts Council and were either awarded a sum or rejected. It seems that there can be no such uniformity now because the fact that RAAs are autonomous has become a recognized position in our post *Glory of the Garden* state. The RAAs believe that there can be harmonization of procedures but not uniformity because:

a) the state of music is different in each region;
b) in response to particular regional needs RAAs have devised particular policies, both overall and on music specifically;
c) RAAs have ways of generating new work and its performance besides commissions, for example by composers in residence schemes.

There can be a check-list regarding procedures but it is clear that there will be no uniformity from region to region because of the individual needs and policies of each RAA. This is perfectly understandable except that it creates the most bizarre anomalies. To take just one example, a composer who happens to have a first performance in one region might be expected to find some of his commission fee himself, while in another region he might be given the full amount or even have it suggested that the commission fee applied for is too low to be considered! I know of cases where figures have been pushed up and down in order that it should become someone else's problem to find the money to fund the commission. (Before the figure of £4,000 was arrived at recently, the cut-off point between the Arts Council and the RAAs was £1,860, a strange sum indeed and open to just that sort of 'political' treatment, where an application is thrown around committee rooms until it finally loses all its relevance.)

Other anomalies exist in the current commissioning procedures. Whereas book publishers and record companies are eligible to make application to receive financial assistance from the Council for 'non-commercial' material, music publishers are not able to qualify for grants to assist them in the preparation and publication of commissioned works funded by the Council. This is just one of the many matters which still need to be resolved in the Arts Council and RAAs commissioning policies.

I am not seeking to lay the blame at any particular door for the current problems regarding commissioning. In fact, having been involved in some of the discussions myself I am hardly clear of suspicion in the accusation of unwieldy bureaucracy creating unnecessary difficulty for the creative artist.

Much could, of course, be achieved, if the Arts Council and RAAs were given substantial increases in funding. One does not need a crystal ball to know that this is unlikely. This sad fact makes it all the more essential that there is clear and informed direction given in the matter of commissioning. Certain vital questions need to be tackled. What is a commission for? Is it merely supporting the composer during a work's composition? If so, would not the award of a bursary be more appropriate? How much should one try and steer composers in a particular direction when commissioning? How much should positive discrimination for or against particular types of works be encouraged?

If there is a moral to all this it is that there are certain times when composers are always right. I am sure that their instincts regarding their unborn music are more to be trusted than the instincts of those who are charged with the formalities of overseeing the comparatively simple task of arranging the payment of commission fees. In the year of 1816 a composer received the following letter:

Dear Mr Schubert,
I wish to protest in the strongest possible manner about your latest composition, which has just been delivered to me. The symphony is all right so far as it goes, but it appears to be incomplete. You have not bothered to finish it.
   Believe me, Mr Schubert, nobody is ever going to listen to an incomplete piece of music, let alone pay good money to do so. Is this some sort of blackmail for increased fees? You have not complained of being underpaid before.
   I am returning the work and I regret that I

shall have to withold payment for it until you have added the final part of the last movement. When that is done I would be glad if you could give the work a title, which is at present lacking.

If I may offer a word of personal advice, Mr Schubert, you must pull yourself together and do better than this. If you cannot be bothered to complete pieces nobody is going to trouble with your music.
Yours etc.

Let us never forget that it is Schubert's name we remember today and not his commissioner. The payer of the piper may indeed call the tune but I would like to hazard a guess that a good many pipers have better tunes on offer if only the circumstances allowed them to play what they really wanted.

For those seeking a composer to commission do not forget to contact the British Music Information Centre and for general advice contact the Composers' Guild. The Guild has a recommended draft commissioning contract. Here are the recommended fee levels for serious music, proposed by The Composers' Guild in association with the Association of Professional Composers. It should be stressed that these figures do not include the cost of preparing and providing performance materials. Such costs are additional and are the commissioner's separate responsibility.

1   Solo/Duo Works (not including works for piano, harp, and keyboard which are rated in category number 2): £60–80 a minute.
2   A Cappella Choral Work or Work for 3–9 Players: £70–120 a minute.
3   Large Chamber Ensemble (10–20 Players): £90–140 a minute.
4   Chamber Orchestra: £130–170 a minute.
5   Orchestral/Choral Works: £160–220 a minute.
6   Electronic Music: £90–120 a minute.
7   Instrumental/Vocal Works with Tape
These should be charged at the rates recommended for the appropriate category of work, plus 50 per cent of the above-quoted rate for preparation of the tape.
8   Opera – Grand or Chamber
This should relate to the recommended fees for orchestral/choral works. If an opera is intended to have three acts of 45 minutes each, a commissioning fee should be commensurate with the comparable length of orchestral/choral music plus an

appropriate amount for producing a piano score. It should be understood that the libretto must be considered separately.

Commissioning bodies

The Arts Council and the RAAs are by far the biggest providers of grants to help with commissioning of new works. For sums under £4,000 the commissioner should approach the RAA in the area in which the work is to be performed. The Arts Council deals only with sums above £4,000 or with works to be premièred outside an RAA area or commissioned for the Contemporary Music Network. The Composers' Guild information sheet on commissions states that in all cases of successful application the composer will receive half the sum immediately, and the other half when the Council or RAA has been informed by the commissioner that the work has been completed. In the event of an unsuccessful application, the composer might suggest an application to a private trust, such as the Vaughan Williams (RVW) Trust (except in the case of London performances) or the Hinrichsen Foundation.

As stated above, policies for the award of commissioning grants and copying costs vary between the Council and RAAs. The current conditions are available from the Music officers at each of the RAAs.

Copying costs

Normally it is the commissioner who makes the claim after all the receipted invoices have been provided. In practice, the Arts Council and RAAs allow the composer to undertake this responsibility. It is acceptable to the Arts Council for the composer to act as his or her own copyist and to submit invoices at the standard Musicians Union rate (though check with the RAAs about this matter).

If there is no award by the Council or RAAs, possible support to these costs might be given by the RVW Trust or SPNM (Francis Chagrin Fund).

The Arts Council of Great Britain,
105, Piccadilly, London W1V 0AU
(Music Department): tel. 01 629 9495.
Scottish Arts Council, 19, Charlotte Square, Edinburgh EH2 4DF (Music Department):
tel. 031 226 6051.

Welsh Arts Council, 9, Museum Place, Cardiff CF1 3NX (Music Department): tel. 0222 394711.

Arts Council of Northern Ireland, 181a, Stranmillis Road, Belfast BT9 5DU (Music Department): tel. 0232 663591.

East Midlands Arts, Mountfields House, Forest Road, Loughborough, Leics. LE11 3HU: tel. 0509 218292.

Eastern Arts Association, 8–9, Bridge Street, Cambridge CB2 1UA: tel. 0223 357596.

Greater London Arts Association, 9 White Lion Street, London N1 9PD: tel. 01 837 8808.

Lincolnshire & Humberside Arts, St Hugh's, 23, Newport, Lincoln LN1 3DN: tel. 0522 33555.

Merseyside Arts, 6, Bluecoat Chambers, School Lane, Liverpool L1 3BX: tel. 051 709 0671/8.

North Wales Association for the Arts, 10, Wellfield House, Bangor, Gwynedd LL57 1ER: tel. 0248 353248.

North West Arts, 12, Harter Street, Manchester M1 6HY: tel. 061 228 3062.

Northern Arts, 10, Osborne Terrace, Newcastle upon Tyne NE2 1NZ: tel 0632 816334.

South East Arts Association, 9–10, Crescent Road, Tunbridge Wells, Kent TN1 2LU: tel. 0892 41666.

South East Wales Arts Association, Victoria Street, Cwmbran, Gwent NP44 3YT: tel. 06333 67530.

South West Arts, Bradninch Place, Gandy Street, Exeter EX4 3LS: tel. 0392 218188.

Southern Arts Association, 19, Southgate Street, Winchester SO23 9EB: tel. 0962 55099.

West Midlands Arts, Brunswick Terrace, Stafford ST16 1BZ: tel. 0785 59231/5.

West Wales Association for the Arts, Dark Gate, Red Street, Carmarthen SA31 1QL: tel. 0267 234248.

Yorkshire Arts Association, Glyde House, Glydegate, Bradford BD5 0BQ: tel. 0274 723051.

Area Arts Associations

Mid Pennine Arts Association, 2, Hammerton Street, Burnley, Lancs. BB11 1NA: tel. 0282 21986/21953.

Fylde Arts Association, Grundy Art Gallery, Queen Street, Blackpool FY1 1PX: tel. 0253 22130.

MICHAEL FINNISSY

Composers in Education: 1

In recent years much of the public funding accorded to performing ensembles in this country has become linked to, and often conditional upon, some sort of educational outlet. On paper the notion seems laudable enough: to inform, promote, and present music (of all kinds, although the bias here is towards contemporary) to a future public while at a young and impressionable age: and certainly anyone who has had contact with children will tell you how receptive they can be when presented with these opportunities. Most of the larger companies and ensembles, such as ENO, Opera North, Scottish Opera, London Contemporary Dance Theatre, London Sinfonietta, and so on, employ a considerably practised staff to handle their educational projects, cover a large sector of the available market, and maintain a good track record.

These schemes, mainly city based, originate from, and are perhaps designed to run concurrently with, earlier initiatives to promote the arts in higher education and the community. During the growth in the number of universities in the 1960s, many of the newly created music departments encouraged composers and performing musicians to be on their staff, as if to add authenticity and glamour, and stave off the bookish theorizing that can replace a vital, if also unstable, living tradition. However, few university music departments continued unconditionally to support musicians once cuts in the education budget appeared; few in any case had enabled them simply to carry on with their own work (Trinity College, Cambridge was and is a notable exception). In most instances the musician in a university environment is expected to 'work for a living', i.e. become involved in curriculum teaching and administration, and not give concerts or compose, although these can be considered as significant sidelines. Employing musicians this way is obviously beneficial to the students, but less so to the musician. Inevitably even the best-prepared teaching schedule, however invigorating at first, stands a good chance of deteriorating after a number of years into dull routine, in turn producing music which is itself as dull and unpalatable as its parent entrenched academicism.

Broader-based community action in the arts nominally arrived with the spread of regional Arts Councils, and a number of 'artists in the community' were appointed. The appointments were often quite ludicrous though, as suitable artists already resident in the areas concerned were overlooked in favour of short-term imports, and the resulting lack of adequate follow through, or long-term liaison with community groups, undermined many of these schemes. Not surprisingly, they seem generally to have been phased out, and replaced by less broadly based, usually educationally biased proposals, or indeed by individual localized commissions.

The issue of 'follow through' in any arts-oriented educational endeavour is the one constantly highlighted by composers. Lack of long-range planning is, unfortunately, an all too frequent component of contemporary arts patronage – representing a reluctance or inability to accept responsibility for, or even foresee the consequence of, its actions – rather as though an agriculturalist were to go into a field with a handful of valuable seeds and simply fling them onto the ground, in the hope that at least some might take root, but lacking either the capacity or the willingness to look after whichever did. Our culture is too multi-faceted and diverse for such lack of care and foresight, particularly in the planning of educational issues: short-term stimulation is most likely to have a merely short-term effect. With the present lack of faith in the entire education system, very few teachers have enough time or sufficient commitment to nurture properly the uneconomical specialist area of the arts. Confusion about what is 'good' in contemporary music is also rampant – token acceptance of funk, jazz, pop, rock, and soul (not to mention the various 'ethnic' musics) is not likely to simplify or clarify this issue. Problems of *what* to teach; or what the basic compositional disciplines are; how to assess music (if at all) as to its quality; and how to provide adequate long-term access to even a representative selection of material via books, sheet-music, records, cassettes, CDs, or videos merely compound these difficulties.

'Follow through' is also recognizable to anyone with a working knowledge of creative disciplines as the *fundamental* ingredient in composition. Composing is what you do with a musical idea, *not* the idea itself. The initiation of ideas is both relatively easy and insignificant – the ability to create a continuity, knowing how to extend and develop the ideas, or even knowing which are most likely to bear fruitful extension, forms the real crux of the matter. Likewise with group-based (as distinct from individual) music education, if we are to progress beyond the 'game-playing' stage that we are currently in, someone will have to recognize and formulate a means of progressing beyond the moment to moment, flash-in-the-pan, supplying of stimuli, to long-range incorporation of education in the arts – or arts into education – and the fully integrated normalization of such a notion in our culture as a whole.

All composers are to some extent educators, even though the quality of their discourse – whether verbal or musical – is not always most profitably directed at children. Surely we should now also regard it as odd that an artist needs to be titled 'in the community' to be regarded as such, or do we still believe that artists dwell in ivory towers or customarily *outside* the community?

I would like to thank six distinguished and highly experienced colleagues for their much-valued ideas in compiling the above digest: Judith Weir, David Bedford, Ian McQueen, Stephen Oliver, Nigel Osborne, and Paul Patterson. As a supplement to the foregoing here is a selection of their thoughts, culled from interviews, but appreciably less altered or mangled by me.

Judith Weir

- Arts events need to be more outgoing, so that there is less need for indoctrination sessions.
- To get to one of the roots of the issue: administrators and musicians also need to be better educated.
- Exploit local needs.
- Maybe we have too low an opinion of the capacity of children to learn, and their own critical sense.
- The composer's concern with education is far more genuine than some administrators.
- Teachers in schools can be resentful of the presence of outside musicians, unless they are very self-confident, because their own work is so undervalued by society in general.
- Often a 'residency' is a means of obtaining cut-price teaching (part-time or fellowship fees for a full-time involvement).

David Bedford

- Music education should start in primary schools, with adventurous teachers, and in parallel with developing writing skills.
- Participation from the students is a necessity in any educational work.
- Younger groups need an evocative text as a stimulus to composition, older groups (11–15) begin to develop curiosity about 'intellectual' levels of music – variation form for example.
- There is the 'barrier' of notation to musical composition, which is not found in other forms of writing or in painting.
- You do have to be a composer to teach composition.

Ian McQueen

- The original material (aspiration) is relatively unimportant, providing it is *clear*, and that there is an awareness of intent.
- Teach economy of gesture, free from 'intellectual' artifice.
- The artist is a living embodiment of Art as a stimulus within society.
- Educational responses have to take place in the real world, however vile that may be. It is essential to retain integrity, and the ability to respond honestly to circumstances and people: the affectation of 'local colour' is not necessary.
- It is important to encourage children to discriminate between sounds.

Stephen Oliver

- There is no point in becoming involved with education, any more than with composing generally, unless you learn from it too.
- I am interested in the question of what is actually *happening* when a performance takes place.
- There is no set way of doing a particular piece.
- After determining some sort of framework for a project, I encourage 'feedback' from the group, from their inventing and composing.
- A one-year working schedule (to produce a

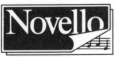

piece for a school) seems practical – initial stimulus, then individual work, then participation sessions and consolidation, finishing up with intensive rehearsals and production.

Nigel Osborne

- In pursuing an evolving culture, a certain competence at the traditional technical apparatus is, of course, necessary – but not as a revered absolute, rather something to control and have power over. Most composition teaching has simply succeeded in sanitizing the creative component.
- There is a danger, especially in becoming involved with community arts projects, of submitting oneself to a confusing plurality of criticism and self-criticism.

- It is important to take ideas beyond the tokenism required by the establishment.
- Working with a group enables you to find a way to say things for which the appetite and space already exists.
- University music can often be a backwash of the compositional subconscious.

Paul Patterson

- Even in a high-powered, some would say 'elitist' establishment, there is the same entrenchment in tradition as in secondary schools; a resistance to, and lack of awareness of, twentieth-century music.
- The initial impetus comes from giving a sense of creating: thereafter 'composing' has to be taught at many different levels.

NICHOLAS BANNAN and MALCOLM SINGER

Composers in Education: 2

The GCSE has moved away from an analytical/historical/theoretical approach towards one which requires creative work, and integrates performance with the other elements of the course. One could draw an analogy with the teaching of English: whereas in the past Music had much in common with the old English Literature approach with its emphasis on set works, the new course will be closer to the spirit of an English Language preparation, with the pupil's own self-expression through the medium central to his/her development of fluency and articulateness. As in the best teaching of English, far from sacrificing all that is tried and sacred in our cultural heritage, the new examination could arguably reinforce traditional values more spontaneously than previous syllabuses which have tended to adhere to the letter rather than the creative spirit of what past composers have achieved, let alone encourage any connections between such 'historical' music and that which is being produced today. The national criteria rightly set great store by the *process* of gaining musical experience – it is not *what* we perform, listen to, or compose that matters, but *how* the pupils develop in these fields. Such a 'value-free' approach obviously frightens some teachers. They should have faith; musical languages have an enormous strength which will hardly dissipate through altering the bases of public examinations. To believe the contrary is to see O Level Music as a sort of pre-Babel orthodoxy, which is neither realistic nor fair to the thousands of schoolchildren who were excluded from studying Music at this level by the nature of the old syllabuses.

How, then, is this new course to be taught? We are concerned here with the issue of composition, so far as it can be separated from the other elements (and this may be an opportune moment to throw in a plea for an increased profile for twentieth-century music in performance). Most teachers only have experience of composition work in the first two or three years of secondary education, and many have not even been giving this. One of the most exciting ingredients of the GCSE is the continuation of such work up to the age of 16, creating a 5-year course in which composing is constantly undertaken and developed. Teachers must be fully able to guide and stimulate such creative work and, most significantly, assess the results both within the course and at its completion. Some teachers have already voiced their hostility to this form of music education, though many are willing to face its implications and welcome any available support. Many have never been taught to compose in their own education, let alone to teach others and will need to undergo a radical change in their perception of the subject if they are to cope. Here, then, is an excellent opportunity for composers (both in 'serious' and other fields, such as jazz) to offer support and stimulus both through helping to train teachers and through working in schools.

It is clear that a place exists for the composer in schools to an extent not common hitherto: his/her field is now a compulsory part of all school music courses which lead to public examination. However, the relationship between visiting composer and teacher, and indeed that between both and the pupils, is complex and must be handled with sensitivity on both sides. (Sadly it is uncommon for Education Authorities to employ specialist composers in the same way that they do brass or woodwind teachers, and full-time work in school is hardly a congenial background for a composer. The development of new schemes to encourage composers to work on permanent contracts, rather than as visiting phenomena, would be of great benefit.) It is all too easy for the 'regular' teacher to feel usurped by the outsider, who may in turn make unrealistic demands on the pupils and teacher. As the composers in the first half of this article imply, it is no easy matter to gauge the time-scale and creative outcome of a developing project. One must remember, too, that this new orientation is the result of an examination, and must involve assessable goals: there is, perhaps regrettably, little room for open-ended experimentation. However well-respected and successful the pioneering work in schools of certain composers and contemporary-music ensembles has been in the past, one must recognize the need for a more consistent and universal policy of support for twentieth-century music and creativity in education than has hitherto been the case.

RICHARD BARRETT
Cornelius Cardew

1 (Auto)biographical

Cornelius Cardew was born on 7 May 1936, in Winchcombe, Gloucestershire. He was a chorister at Canterbury Cathedral from 1943 to 1950, and from 1953 to 1957 studied at the Royal Academy of Music. It seems that his official studies there (composition with Howard Ferguson, piano with Percy Waller) turned out to be less important to him than the opportunity to study, support, play, and learn from the contemporary European avant-garde, which became a strong influence on his early work (no doubt to the bemusement and/or annoyance of the predominant conservatism at the Academy). Having received a RAM scholarship to study electronic music in Cologne in 1957–8, Cardew met Karlheinz Stockhausen, with whom he worked as assistant from 1958 to 1960 and 'collaborated' on the score of *Carré*. According to Stockhausen, 'I left the independent working-out of composition plans to him. Our common experiences have shown how such collaboration might be further developed.'[1] Cardew later wrote 'This score ... would be the score of a piece for four orchestras by Karlheinz Stockhausen and no mistake about it.'[2] Stockhausen pursued what he saw as a collaborative line of development (*Ensemble* (1967), *Musik für ein Haus*, and *Aus den sieben Tagen* (1968), etc.) without at any time denying the centrality of his own personality, finally coming out in favour of promoting a 'new serving mentality'[3] in his associates.

Having begun in the late 1950s to absorb the ideas emanating from the American experimental movement (primarily John Cage and David Tudor) and its genuine attempt to think about and work with such unquestioned (in Europe) musical areas as the composer/performer relationship, the role of notation, the composition of other than the 'sounding result', etc., Cardew began to react against the doctrinaire serialists on the European scene. As a profoundly humanist musician (this quality becomes a constant factor behind what may seem to constitute several radical changes of direction subsequently), he was attracted by the experiments of composers like Cage, Wolff, and Bussotti who in their different ways invited the performers of their music to take an active part in the process of musical realization. The presence of a performer like David Tudor was certainly a catalyst for this development, since composers needed to have the faith that such openness on their part would be constructive (i.e. the performer making real, musical decisions). Boulez and Stockhausen, together with most European composers, treated the idea of the performer's choice as no more than an interesting technical device; Cardew saw what it was really about – music as a collaborative phenomenon in the true sense.

On his return to Britain at the beginning of the 1960s, then, Cardew had placed himself at several removes from the musical establishment. His major work of this period, *Treatise* (1963–7), is to an extent a product of and a reaction to his enforced living conditions at the time – earning a living as a graphic artist. 'Psychologically the existence of the piece is fully explained by the situation of a composer who is not in a position to make music.'[4] It might thus be said that *Treatise*, consisting of 193 pages of undefined, sometimes quasi-notational graphics, is not music but a substitute for music (but what would *that* be?) and also obviously represents an interest in graphic invention as an end in itself. I shall return to the subject of this work, which must be the most introverted and personal in the whole of Cardew's output, but which paradoxically led to his involvement in the least introverted area of music-making: free improvisation, with his joining the group AMM in 1966, consisting at that time of the ex-jazz musicians Lou Gare, Eddie Prevost, Keith Rowe, and Laurence Sheaff.

Towards the end of the 60s, Cardew became important as a teacher of music, both at the RAM (at which his first pupil, Christopher Hobbs, was his *only* one for some time; the Academy had not changed that much in the 10 years since Cardew himself studied there) and at Morley College, where he had the opportunity to attract and work with numbers of like-minded people. His most important work, *The Great Learning* (1968–71) is the work of a composer who *is* in a position to make music. By the time it was complete, the Scratch Orchestra, a large collective of musicians, artists, performers of all kinds both trained and untrained, had been in existence for several years and was about to begin its traumatic process of politicization which was to lead Cardew's work into a new phase and his activities into a different arena; namely his concern for the class struggle.

By the time of Cardew's DAAD scholarship to work in Berlin for a year in 1973 he was trying to undo all the work he had put into producing and publicizing the avant-garde music of the 50s and the experimentalism of the 60s, both his own work and that of others, because his critical approach to music now had as its prime criterion the relevance and appropriateness of a work to the revolutionary liberation of the working classes. When invited by the BBC the year before to write and present a talk introducing a performance of *Refrain* (1959) by his ex-colleague Stockhausen, Cardew produced the text 'Stockhausen Serves Imperialism' – later collected with other musical/political writings in a book of the same title[5] – in which the work of the avant-garde is subjected to examination on Marxist–Leninist–Maoist principles. The same process was applied to Cage and the experimentalists, and to Cardew's own previous work.

Not that Cardew was losing interest in composition during this time; he was actively involved until the end of his life in the process of evolving a music which *would* serve the interests of the working-class revolution, and this process, while remaining unresolved at his death, did indeed produce a great deal of music worthy of his unique musicality. One may speculate on his eventual contribution to music in this country had he lived. In the autumn of 1981 he began a course in analysis at King's College, London, in order to familiarize himself with historical techniques, the better to 'make the past serve the present'. In November of that year, a vaguely familiar-looking figure distributing political leaflets at the refectory of King's College (where I was studying at the time) turned out to be Cardew. There was a brief conversation of little consequence; my own political awareness was nothing to speak of at the time. Several weeks later I heard that he had been killed by a hit-and-run driver on 13 December, near his home in Leyton, East London. Half-way through the next term I left the College, for reasons summed up by an attempt to organize an afternoon session of improvisation at the music department, which I was the only person to attend.

In 1984, taking part in the first complete performance of *The Great Learning*,[6] I began to realize the unique importance of this work and its implications, resumed a commitment to improvisatory musics, began a composition (to date unfinished) to be dedicated to Cardew, as a gesture not of nostalgia but solidarity. I expect that if Cardew knew what I was doing he would accuse me also of serving imperialism; I am trying very hard to do no such thing.

I began work on these notes in 1985, at first intending to request interviews and/or opinions from colleagues of Cardew. I eventually decided against this: knowing of the work in hand towards documentation and appraisal being carried out by John Tilbury, one of Cardew's most authoritative and faithful collaborators (as well as a major influence on Cardew's own politicization), any attempt by myself would be incomplete and redundant. What follows is a collection of reactions and reflections by a composer (painfully) aware of the responsibility of *all* composers to attempt to come to terms with the issues raised by Cardew's work in all its manifestations.

2 Piano

If I begin with Cardew's piano music, which spans his entire career and might be said to be the least radical (i.e. experimental) area of his work, this is because the not inconsiderable literature on Cardew frequently gives a view of him (merely) as a 'man of ideas', rather than a composer of *music* whose qualities need no moral support from their conceptual infrastructure, and which may be judged on the same level as any music by composers less concerned than he was with the nature and status of themselves and their work.

The piano music is the work of an accomplished pianist: anyone who heard Cardew in his earlier days as an exponent of the newest music would testify to this, and he has left eloquent and powerful recordings, with Janos Negyesy, of the four Ives violin sonatas[7] which confirm such a view. As a composer for his own instrument, he shows ever-renewed fascination with its sonorous possibilities, whatever changes his style underwent, inviting comparison with another English composer-pianist, Michael Finnissy. In the piano works of both, a strong and continuing source of ideas is experience of the instrument itself, and both eventually assimilated both the post-war avant-garde pianism and that of the nineteenth-century virtuosi into their scheme of things, albeit in entirely different ways. Whereas Stockhausen, for example, designed his piano pieces as compositional études, 'drawings' for more finished and expressive works, Cardew and Finnissy project through the medium something very basic about their musical personalities; the piano is somehow at the heart of their respective aesthetics, a prime contributory factor to my conviction that they are the two most important writers for the piano that this country has produced.

Cardew's Piano Sonata No. 3 (1958) shows these pianistic qualities to a greater extent than his previous works; the Second Sonata, for example, bears the stamp of Boulez's *Structures I* for two pianos (of which Cardew and Richard Rodney Bennett had given the first British performance, at the RAM) in its astringent use of integral-serial methods. The third, however, despite displaying just as abstract a musical skeleton, breaks into streams of grace notes which glitter across the keyboard as subsequently completed works of Stockhausen (e.g. *Klavierstücke VI* and *X*) were to do: a *rapprochement* has been achieved between serial aridity and an irrepressible need to use the piano as more than an analytical projector of structure. This sonata is followed by the *Two Books of Study for Pianists* (also 1958) (Ex. 1) which is separated from the earlier work by the 'American experience'. The ideas which generated Stockhausen's *Klavierstück XI* and Boulez's Third Sonata have already been more fully appreciated by Cardew, who, stemming as he did from a virtually negligible sense of indigenous musical tradition, was perhaps more susceptible to take a path contrary to the European mainstream. Not that Cardew was now slavishly following the Cageian line of abstraction from sound during composition – the *Two Books* define not a precise musical object but, in Cardew's own term, a 'musizierweisse',[8] a mode of music-making, information which, imparted by means of the score to the interpreters, enables them to understand and operate within the limits which constitute the piece. The definition of such limits in exact accordance with the performer- and perception-related aspects of the proposed music becomes a more and more important compositional concern of Cardew's through the 60s, culminating in *The Great Learning* as a supreme example of just enough information to create a musical identity for a work, without compromising the responsibility placed on a performer to think out and contribute his or her *own* music. In the *Two Books*, however, and the piano music which follows, these ideas are seen in terms specifically of a pianist (or pianists) and, again in contradistinction to Cage, the 'taste and memory' of that pianist, the vast area of connotation around the fact of *being* a pianist. The next work for piano, *February Pieces* (1959–61), focuses further in on 'pianistic psychology', rushing headlong and irrationally through a wide scale of 'receivedness', figurational familiarity, expressive disjointedness. The process of working *with* the piano continues through the *Three Winter Potatoes* (1961–5), the first of which is actually a realization of the cryptic symbols constituting *Octet 61*, thus emphasizing Cardew's view of the piano as a theatre of, as it were, *concrete* music-making. The symbols are transformed into a more fully-notated

Example 1

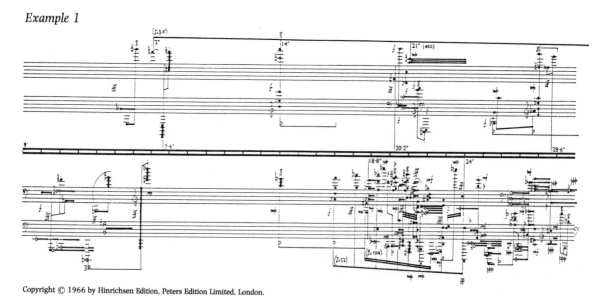

music which is not only psychologically consistent (at least within the framework of aleatoric fragmentation) but also characteristically pianistic in its deployment of the gestural suggestions. A further 'concretization' which, at least as far as its performance history to date is concerned, relates to the piano, is *Volo Solo* (1965). This was written as a 'virtuoso piece' for John Tilbury, although it may be performed, omitting pitches outside the available range, on any instrument: it consists of 'the entire formal scheme of *Treatise* transliterated into well-tempered pitches';[9] most aspects of interpretation are free except that each of the swarms of pitches, separated by gaps, which constitute the score are to be performed at a (subjectively) reckless pace. 'The instrument' Cardew wrote, 'should seem to be breaking apart.'[10] Ex. 2, from the preface to the score, shows an excerpt in which the pitch-range of a bassoon (as an arbitrary example) is delineated by horizontal lines, and then the same excerpt in a hypothetical performing version for that instrument. Despite all this, the fact that the piano is the only readily-available instrument which can play all the notated material, as well as being the instrument most able to account for the piece's manipulation of the 'as fast as possible' instruction by rapid variations, i.e. the extent to which the music lies under the hands (however fortuitous this may be), marks *Volo Solo* as a piano piece at heart. In a similar way *Memories of You* (1964), a homage to Cage and especially to his *Concert for Piano and Orchestra* (1957–8), could have been written with virtually any instrument in mind, but in fact consists of diagrammatical instructions as to where in relation to a piano the (undefined) sounds should occur. The title of this piece may relate to Cage. It may also refer to the piano itself, to which Cardew, at least as a composer, bade a temporary farewell during the *Treatise*/AMM period. The attitude of the work to the instrument is ambiguous: the three sound-sources A, B, and C may actually involve the participation of the piano, or equally, may be connected with it only by proximity, as if Cardew's journey into musical experiment had progressed beyond the point where piano music is possible.

Once Cardew, in the early 70s, had decided to deny himself the bourgeois individualism of such eccentricity, the piano once again becomes the centre of his musical activity, not least through being virtually omnipresent in potential performing spaces. In the *Piano Album 1973*, brief and uncomplicated melodies (mostly Irish and revolutionary Chinese in origin) are adapted in an equally simple, almost naïve, but profoundly pianistic manner. *Father Murphy* (Ex. 3) has this characteristic lack of sophistication but is one of the most hauntingly emotional pieces one could wish to hear: its sparse gestures spring out of the piano with great freshness and poignancy. The *Thälmann Variations* of 1974, named for the chairman of the German Communist Party who was interned in 1933 and executed in 1944 by the Nazis, is equally inventive with piano sonority, from the harp-like broken chords at the beginning onwards, but suffers, together with other examples of avant-garde or experimental composers adopting a melodic/tonal style (Stockhausen, Takahashi, etc.) of being harmonically and formally rather clumsy, seemingly disjointed when it should be mellifluous and vice versa. Perhaps this clumsiness was deliberate. In any case, Cardew's last compositions for piano, *Boolavogue* (for two pianos) and *We Sing for the Future*, both 1981, show a greater integration of the procedures of tonal music, especially of the baroque and earlier. The latter piece involves strict contrapuntal working, and both use folk-music or folk-like material

Example 2

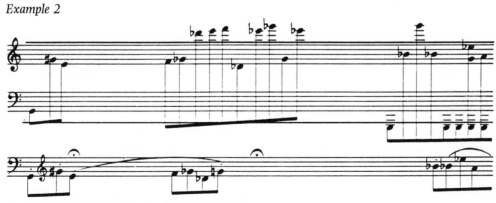

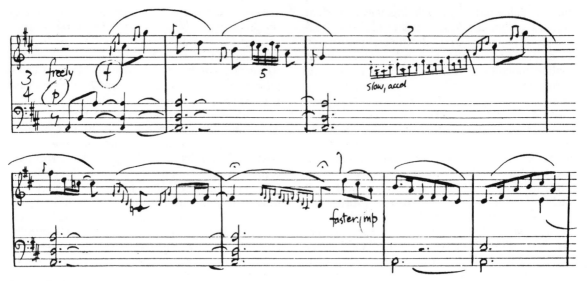

Example 3

(much as did their models in earlier music) for its innate characteristics and for the (partly submerged) emotional effect of its subject matter. (Both types of impact were certainly in evidence when John Tilbury, announcing *Boolavogue* at a London concert during the miners' strike of 1984–5, mentioned its performance in mining country shortly before – one of the tunes used in the piece is *The Blackleg Miner*.) The road towards a reconsideration of sophistication in Cardew's music had begun by 1981; with these two pieces we shall have to content ourselves with only the beginning.

3 Improvising

Treatise may on one level be a reaction to Cardew's prevailing circumstances, but there is a great deal more to it than that: any examination of the score reveals it as a valuable contribution to the discussion of notation, its purposes and priorities, as well as a highly accomplished and beautiful piece of design, and an enigmatic but powerful stimulus to music production.

The score itself is a complex, quasi-developmental treatment of 67 elements[11] which generates, upon silent reading, the impression of a large-scale, almost symphonic, musical span, with areas of relaxation and areas of climax (notably the build-up to the enormous burst of black circles on page 133, (Ex. 4) which never fails to evoke a reaction hardly different from that of a particularly cataclysmic passage in 'real' music). Several of

Cardew's more explicitly-notated works (they could hardly be less) of the 60s are 'realizations' of parts of this massive score: *Volo Solo* has already been mentioned; *Bun No. 2* for orchestra (1964) is another example, and there may be others which Cardew did not advertise as such. Nevertheless, *Treatise* has become a work to be realized as it is, usually in the form of more or less premeditated improvisation. Rather than representing an alternative mode of realization to the ones mentioned above, this exemplifies Cardew's hope that 'in playing *Treatise* the performer will give of his own music in response to my music, which is the score itself'.[12] But as Tilbury says, 'its visual impact disconcertingly puts most performances of it in the shade'.[13] I have experienced myself the exquisite frustration which results from attempting to create sounds as an interpretation of the score: any consistent treatment of the elements on a given page is inevitably contradicted by the presence of one or more contradictory features. The resultant impression is that there *is* a sonic analogue to what is on the page, that it will remain forever just out of reach, but that something about *Treatise* consistently makes musical sense.

It was of course impossible for Cardew to pursue this line; like Wittgenstein in the *Tractatus logico-philosophicus*, from which Cardew's title is derived, he had said everything possible given a certain view of the field of enquiry. The only logical step after the experience of 'performing' *Treatise* was for Cardew to enter more fully the world of free improvisation, which he did upon joining AMM. I

Example 4

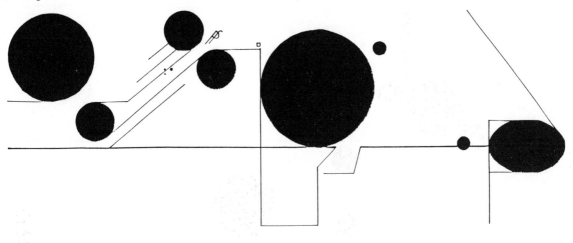

130

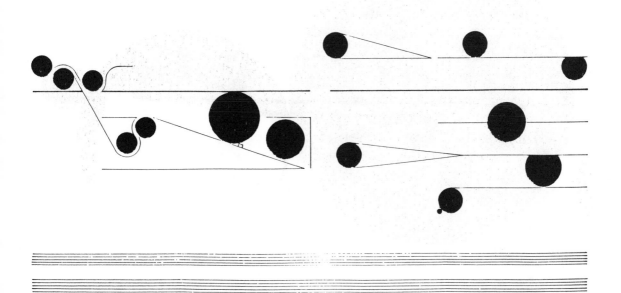

131

25

(Example 4 cont.)

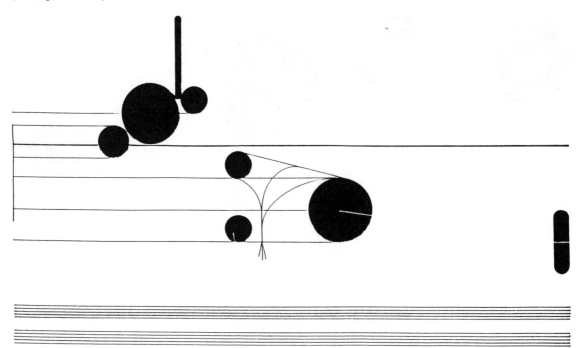

132

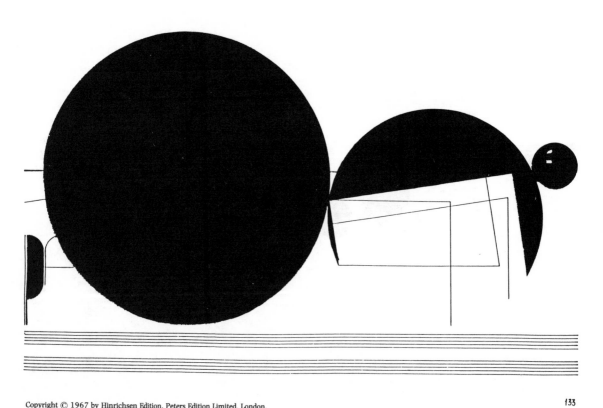

133

do not propose to dwell upon the work of AMM as such, since Cardew, it should be remembered, was in no sense its leader or even a *primus inter pares*, but it is important in the light of his work as a whole to attempt to appreciate what he *meant* by improvisation, which was not exactly what a jazz player or non-Western musician would make of the word. In *Towards an Ethic of Improvisation*, published in the *Treatise Handbook*, Cardew significantly adopts the method of the *later* Wittgenstein, who in *Philosophical Investigations*, for example, 'has *abandoned theory*, and all the glory that theory can bring on a philosopher (or musician), in favour of an illustrative technique'.[14] Although AMM music was generally quite individual and recognizable, Cardew in no way gives a 'recipe' for it, confining himself to a list of 'virtues a musician can develop': simplicity, integrity, selflessness, forbearance, preparedness, identification with nature, and acceptance of death. What then takes place musically is nothing more nor less than the result of a group of people applying these precepts in each other's company: 'AMM *is* their sounds (as ignorant of them as one is about one's own nature).'[15] What improvisation meant, then, was an activity as unforced and central to a musical life as respiration to organic life. His subsequent work on *The Great Learning* was an attempt to make this realization more available and accessible to those without years to invest in acquiring a 'musical state of being'.

During Cardew's Maoist years and the concentration on a social-realist idiom, the exhilarating but inevitably somewhat closed activity of free improvisation was discontinued in favour of music which could communicate its revolutionary message without the barrier to understanding created by the experimental ethos. In retrospect this can be seen as a temporary over-reaction, upon becoming belatedly aware of the 'irrelevance' of contemporary art music and its institutions in general; once again it wasn't temporary enough, and Cardew's projected reunion with AMM to perform *Treatise* in 1982 was prevented from taking place.

4 The Great Learning

I have mentioned above that one of Cardew's most important achievements in the field of experimental music is that of an appropriate mix of freedom and discipline in the compositions, such that, on the one hand, the performer is fruitfully involved in discovering his or her own musical resources, and on the other hand, the listener is presented with a definite and satisfying musical experience. *The Great Learning*, in its attempt to create such situations in the context of a larger performing body than was usual in experimental work previous to its conception (which is of course intimately related to that of the Scratch Orchestra and Cardew's class at Morley College), is intended as a model of quasi-social relationships between, in this case, performers (and between them and their audience).

Cardew had been interested in the Confucian writings for some years: the *Treatise Handbook* contains a reference dated March 1963 to Ezra Pound's translation of the *Ta Hsio* (i.e., the Great Learning),[16] and his eventual setting of its seven paragraphs, at least in its most familiar and published form, uses that translation. Pound was interested in making poetry out of the bare outlines supplied by the Chinese ideograms, and his translation contains numerous instances of an alternative figurative utterance alongside a more exact rendering: thus in paragraph 5, 'given the extreme knowable points, the inarticulate thoughts were defined with precision' is supplemented by 'the sun's lance coming to rest on the precise spot verbally'. This device of Pound's, to be found throughout his translations (as well as his original poetry) no doubt renders the text more amenable to the conception of musical settings or analogues: a more accurate translation of the above would be 'thoughts having been made sincere, minds were rectified'.[17] Pound was searching in Confucius for a world order based upon social discipline and a reverence for culture, which he eventually believed he had found in Mussolini's Fascism; Cardew's search for a model of collective responsibility (in music) also evolved through an absorption with Confucius, but one which at this stage critically ignored the reactionary social content of the *Ta Hsio*, seeing in it only his bourgeois ideal of order in, for example, the end of paragraph 5:

> Having attained this self-discipline, they set their own houses in order. Having order in their own homes, they brought good government to their own states. And when their states were well governed, the empire was brought into equilibrium.

His concern for 'equilibrium' caused him to ignore the importance and connotations (to Pound and to Confucius) of the word 'empire'.

Subsequent to Cardew's espousal of Communism, new translations of the texts were made (in 1972) which attempted to steer their emphasis towards populism; in paragraph 1, for instance, 'it

[The Great Learning] is rooted in watching with affection the way people grow', becomes 'The Great Learning is rooted in love for the broad masses of the people', and so on. Cardew also stipulated that, in the 1972 Proms performance of parts of this version, banners bearing revolutionary slogans (e.g. 'A revolution is not a dinner party, it is an insurrection, an act of violence by which one class overthrows another') were to be displayed. Needless to say, this was prevented by the BBC: in any case, by the time Cardew wrote his critical essay on the piece in 1974,[18] his attitude towards it had changed once more. He now repudiated any attempt (e.g. by Pound, by Christian missionaries in China, by himself) to warp the Confucian text into a confirmation of 'pet ideas' and reverted to the original version, so that a performance would reveal its class character and ideological content intact and hold it up to be criticized, in the interests of enlightening its audience by disengagement, the realization that what is happening on stage (in *all* its aspects) is an exposé of techniques used by the ruling class for the purpose of institutional reaction. Whether or not one accepts the validity of this or any other mode of performance of the work, its stature as a musically successful large-scale composition, as it is, is difficult to deny. Moreover, it is fundamentally based around Pound's translation to the extent that to use any other ends up being inappropriate as well as compromising.

The Great Learning is a summation of practically everything Cardew had learned about the workings of music. It is possible to see traces of the abstract serialist composer in the way it is organized around its text, not only in the sense of analogizing musical situations and processes from it, but also in that the text is, as it were, used economically in the generation of seemingly empirical material. Two examples: firstly, the graphic notations for whistles (paragraph 1; Ex. 5) and gueros (paragraph 4) are derived from the strokes of the Chinese characters making up that part of the text; secondly, the numbers of repetitions of words and phrases in paragraph 7 are the numbers of strokes used to form the characters of those words or phrases. There are many other examples of this arcane kind of derivation to be found in the score. The composer of 'inspirational' notations as in the *Two Books of Study*, and then *Treatise, Schooltime Compositions*, etc., is found in the organ parts of paragraphs 1 and 4, which invite the organist to elaborate imaginatively on a fairly sparse (staff-based) notation, and also the 'Number Score' and 'Action Score' of paragraph 5, which are points of departure for flights of irrationality (however 'disciplined'). The 'Ode Machines' of paragraph 5 and the vocal part of paragraph 2 also point forward to Cardew's later interest in an uncomplicated tonal idiom. The score as a whole, above all, is a frequently exuberant (and almost encyclopaedic) celebration of the possibilities inherent in a collective like the Scratch Orchestra, a theatre of action in which as many as a hundred performers are invited to discover and contribute (in a decisive manner) their personal and social musicality.

In paragraph 1, apart from an opening passage on clicking pebbles and an almost fully-notated organ prelude (the most 'traditional' notation in the whole work), an alternation is set up between complete statements of the text by the speaking chorus, and interpretations by successive soloists of a passage in ideogram-derived notation, performed on a 'whistle' while those elsewhere in the batting order contribute to a chordal whistling drone. In the 1984 performance, as no doubt originally, the word 'whistle' was variously interpreted as a referee's whistle, swanee whistle, recorder mouthpiece, etc., which in the event gave quite an exhaustive view of what different renditions of the same notation are possible, from 'avant-garde' virtuosity with multiphonics to perverse (and silent) slapstick. The austere repetitions of the text ('. . . clarifying the way wherein the intelligence increases through the process of looking straight into one's own heart and acting on the results . . .') produce Confucius's 'perfect equity' in their balance with such latitude.

Paragraph 2 sounds very different, and also

Example 5

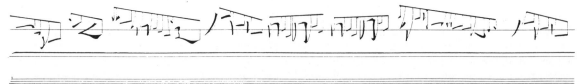

involves the performers in a different way. The text is sung five times through by several groups of singers, each with a leader (to indicate their entries and provide the pitch) and a drummer. The volume generated by the drumming (of 26 repeated rhythmic cells, in an order left free to each drummer) creates an obstacle to the voices making themselves heard, especially as each repetition of the text transposes the sung (pentatonic) melody, each note occupying one long breath, up by a semitone so that the singers, by the end, not only have had to sustain maximum volume for around an hour, but also, to varying degrees, must reach for difficult high notes. Cardew in his instructions allows for octave transpositions in such cases, but it would seem appropriate in view of the explicitly challenging nature of the piece to 'attempt the impossible' or, in the words of the text, to 'keep one's head in moments of danger'. In his note for the commercial recording of paragraph 2, Cardew stresses the feeling of failure engendered by singing the piece, which is mirrored in the dissolution of coherence in the singing as the groups fall out of time with one another while at the end the drum-rhythms are intended to move *towards* coherence once the singing has ended. Like most of *The Great Learning*, then, the situation created in this piece is defined in such a way as to negate any advantage in the possession (or lack) of musical training in its performers.

Paragraph 3 is more concerned with defining an overall sound than a performance attitude. The text ('things have root and branch . . .') is exemplified by a number of bass instruments (10 is suggested) playing slow ascending scales from a low Ab which is returned to as a drone; Cardew suggests several examples of scales (Ab major, ascending fourths, etc.) although instrumentalists are encouraged to invent their own. When this texture has been set up, the words are sung to any note of a three-note chord until this too has been established, whereupon the singers move individually to pitches they can hear (without transposition) from the ascending instrumental scales. This process occurs three times, each with a new chord: the chords are A major, Eb minor, and C (no third). After this, a freer treatment of the material occurs for a duration determined only by the wishes of the vocalists (or a prearranged signal). The effect of these processes is not, as in paragraph 2, of dissolution but of a definite initial situation giving rise to a proliferating (harmonic) richness, as close to 'absolute' music as is attained in *The Great Learning*.

Paragraph 4, again, is more outgoing, and

has the character of a ritual or processional. The organ part here is more schematic, and may also be realized in part by groups of homogeneous-sounding instruments; its seven sections correspond to those of the text, which are set to a canon in which the vocalists shout the syllables singly in rhythmic unison while striking a cushion or similar object with a long 'wand'. The canon, each part one very slow beat (i.e. 5–10 seconds) behind the previous one, passes down a long line of seated vocalists which snakes through the performing space. With a sufficient number of performers the end of the line is a considerable time behind the beginning; not only does the text pass slowly down it (reflecting the logical train of thought in the text, on the subject of setting up 'good government'), but so do the graphic passages, this time interpreted on gueros, between sentences. This canonic verse/interlude structure is succeeded by a coda in which each vocalist, after finishing his or her part, recapitulates all seven guero passages without a break. The piece thus ends with the gradual thinning-out of a chorus of gueros, its length dictated primarily by the number of performers, like paragraph 1. It seems to generate in performance just that quasi-mystical ambience that Cardew later criticized, which the optional improvised vocal solos do not do much to dispel. However, the difficulty of maintaining the extremely slow tempo, in the face of a great deal of interference from organ and gueros, certainly contributes to a suitably ceremonial, even funereal, attitude in performance, and eventually a feeling of great freedom and relief having come out at the other side, when the procession, of sounds rather than people, has vanished into the distance.

The idea of discipline followed by release is exploited more fully in paragraph 5, in which a complex juxtaposition and superimposition of more or less disciplined action is followed by a group improvisation of similar length with no instruction other than 'a dense forest that presents no obstacle to the mind or eye (or other sense)'. The improvisational situation here is a quite unique experience; although the heart of paragraph 5 is contained in the words 'they disciplined themselves' and the restrictions of the first half are intended as a preparatory action for it, the aforementioned release could equally give rise to the opposite of discipline. I am not sure whether this did or did not happen in the 1984 performance, in which the improvisation was seemingly anarchic and contained much that had little to do with what had happened previously, or indeed with music. The conglomeration of a dumb show in sign language (laboriously memorized), improvised soloing, text-recitations, the Action and Number scores, seven verbally-described 'compositions', and ten fully-notated but unsynchronized vocal parts (the Ode Machines) seem to collapse the four days of isolated and silent preparation specified in 'Goldstaub' from Stockhausen's *Aus den sieben Tagen* (1968) into one hour (by no means isolated or silent): during the improvisation one is more aware of the freedom to do or play *anything* than the exhortation to act responsibly. Paragraph 5 is significantly described by Cardew as his 'view of the composition of the [Scratch] orchestra as it now exists [1971], with its high level of differentiation of actions and functions'[19] – also with its eventually destructive internal contradictions.

Paragraph 6 preserves the scheme of adjacent paragraphs contrasting with one another (although they were not conceived as being performed all together, for obvious reasons). In the instructions it is suggested that sound-sources used elsewhere in *The Great Learning* would be suitable: stones, whistles, speech, song, gueros, etc., but these are not individually specified. This piece requires intense listening by participants, of the kind that characterizes the ideal of free

improvisation: they proceed independently through the piece but must frequently wait for (usually unconsciously-given) cues from the others, or from the environment. Some sounds, too, may be 'heard' rather than 'made'; thus any sound which occurs during performance is not only to be understood as part of it (as in Cage) but is drawn into each individual's performance. The element of 'discipline' is paramount here; it is seldom possible for anyone but the individual to tell where he or she is in the score, let alone whether it is being followed 'accurately' or not.

This is not true of paragraph 7 (Ex. 6 quotes the piece in full) which is an astonishing example of the minimum of instructions giving rise to music of strong identity and direction, although the process of harmonic attenuation from the initial dense dissonance (from all of the performers choosing a pitch randomly and independently) is much quicker, and a kind of equilibrium reached at a higher harmonic density, than might appear likely from the way the score describes it.[20] There seems to be an inherent tendency for the situation initially set up to produce a 'beautiful', diatonically-based harmony from the short-lived chromatic/microtonal opening, even (or especially?) for those with untrained voices. For the listener to a

Example 6

The Great Learning, paragraph 7

→ sing 8	IF
sing 5	THE ROOT
sing 13 (f 3)	BE IN CONFUSION
sing 6	NOTHING
sing 5 (f 1)	WILL
sing 8	BE
sing 8	WELL
sing 7	GOVERNED
hum 7	
→ sing 8	THE SOLID
sing 8	CANNOT BE
sing 9 (f2)	SWEPT AWAY
sing 8	AS
sing 17 (f 1)	TRIVIAL
sing 6	AND
sing 8	NOR
sing 8	CAN
sing 17 (f 1)	TRASH
sing 8	BE ESTABLISHED AS
sing 9 (f 2)	SOLID
sing 5 (f 1)	IT JUST
sing 4	DOES NOT
sing 6 (f 1)	HAPPEN
hum 3 (f 2)	
→ speak 1	MISTAKE NOT CLIFF FOR
MORASS AND TREACHEROUS BRAMBLE	

NOTATION

→ The leader gives a signal and all enter concertedly at the same moment. The second of these signals is optional; those wishing to observe it should gather to the leader and choose a new note and enter just as at the beginning (see below).

"sing 9(f2) SWEPT AWAY" means: sing the words "SWEPT AWAY" on a length-of-a-breath note (syllables freely disposed) nine times; the same note each time; of the nine notes two (any two) should be loud, the rest soft. After each note take in breath and sing again.

"hum 7" means: hum a length-of-a-breath note seven times; the same note each time; all soft.

"speak 1" means: speak the given words in steady tempo all together, in a low voice, once (follow the leader).

PROCEDURE

Each chorus member chooses his own note (silently) for the first line (IF eight times). All enter together on the leader's signal. For each subsequent line choose a note that you can hear being sung by a colleague. It may be necessary to move to within earshot of certain notes. The note, once chosen, must be carefully retained. Time may be taken over the choice. If there is no note, or only the note you have just been singing, or only a note or notes that you are unable to sing, choose your note for the next line freely. Do not sing the same note on two consecutive lines.

Each singer progresses through the text at his own speed. Remain stationary for the duration of a line; move around only between lines.

All must have completed "hum 3(f2)" before the signal for the last line is given. At the leader's discretion this last line may be omitted.

complete performance (as well as a performer), paragraph 7 not only sums up, in its text, the philosophy of the whole work, but also finally reaches a 'point of rest' in its slow, enveloping, totally vocal music which forms an apt conclusion.

It would be difficult to accept paragraph 7, and much else in *The Great Learning*, in a spirit of alienation, whether participating or listening, however one may react to Cardew's own eventual appraisal of it as 'inflated rubbish'[21] and however ambivalent one may feel about its original philosophical aims. It is unfortunate that he did not feel able to use his abilities to organize music in this way in the service of more valid ideological goals, but he had his own reasons for this which I shall attempt to examine in the next and last section.

5 Socialist Music?

I have already touched upon the reasons why Cardew felt his embrace of revolutionary politics precluded any further pursuit of the many developments his music had undergone by 1971; a more important question remains – having accepted that all of a composer's actions are to be tested in the light of their relevance to the furtherance of socialism, and that it is not enough merely to change society gradually but necessary to plan for its overthrow, what is a composer to do next? I do not intend here to offer reasons why composers, or anyone else, should adopt such values; firstly for reasons of space, secondly because it could be and has been explained far more forcefully and succinctly than I would ever manage, and thirdly because the matter is to some degree at least self-evident, and is becoming more so.

Reading Cardew's *Stockhausen Serves Imperialism*, as it grinds on through endless restatements of ideological rhetoric, however soundly based, eventually gives an impression of great bleakness, a dissonance with the optimistic aim of revolution and a new society. At the outset he states that not only is the avant-garde and experimental music of his time worthless because its ideological influence (which is the true end-product of an artist's work, as opposed to the artwork being in some way an end in itself) is irrelevant to the class struggle, but also that (therefore) the book itself is worthless, except in as much as it is a necessary exorcism for those like Tilbury and himself who, unlike the working class, *have* in the past been strongly influenced by artistic modernity.

It became obvious to Cardew that asking the question framed by Mao, 'whom do we serve, what class do we support?', produced the answer that his activity as a composer, as an improviser with AMM, and even as a member of the Scratch Orchestra, much as it may attempt a socialization of music, actually played into the hands of the ruling class and its cultural institutions, thus losing any radical impact it may have had in theory. The politicization of music must be re-thought, the solution lying in *integrating* with the working class rather than either cheering it on from the sidelines or lecturing it from above, however one may thus cut oneself off from existing modes of dissemination. (It might be said that Cardew, having achieved some degree of public profile, was in an artificially good position to make this move.) The idea that music somehow stands outside the realities of the class system is an illusion; therefore the *style* of an engaged socialistic music should be one which is accessible, here and now, to the working people. But what style is that? Cardew's own background as a composer now begins to show itself when discussing the lack of criteria for criticizing modern music:

> By comparison with the effectiveness, wholesomeness, emotion, satisfaction, delight, inspiration and stimulus that we . . . derive from Beethoven, Brahms and the rest, modern music (with very few exceptions) is footling, unwholesome, sensational, frustrating, offensive and depressing.

Although he adds in a footnote (written some time after the main text) that the attractions of bourgeois classical music will fade with the onset of revolution, it is clear that he is making certain assumptions regarding the accessibility of 'Beethoven, Brahms and the rest' to working-class people which might be contested. And if its attractions do fade (say they exist), will this not also be true of the compositions of Cardew and the rest which are in a similar style? And what will the world be left with then? Certainly not popular commercial music. And what are the 'few exceptions' in modern music which *are* effective, wholesome, and so on? Neither in 1974, when the book was published, nor at any time during the seven years remaining to him, did Cardew come near resolving these problems. The number of people whose political awareness and commitment were stirred by his later music must be very small, as must the number who actually had the opportunity of hearing any of it, in comparison with the size of its intended audience. Nevertheless, he continued to work in this direction with single-mindedness and even optimism, and it is my conviction that so must everyone else concerned with the production of music and its relationship with people (if it has none, then it is worthless by anyone's standards), Cardew's work begs a question to which there seems to be no answer, except the principle that musical problems are obviously not as important as political problems.

If working-class people are not in a position of awareness to accept any music in the service of socialism except the inevitable patronage offered by composers like the later Cardew, working in a deliberately simplified and banal idiom, then this is the fault of the processes of exploitation and stultification dealt out by the ruling classes to serve *their* interests. It is not good enough to assume that people who are expected to make rational and informed political decisions are at the same time incapable of being rational and informed about the culture of their projected society. It is unfortunate that most people are not in a position to come into contact, let alone sympathize, with radical musical ideas.

6 List of works

This is a provisional catalogue, pending completion of work by the Cornelius Cardew Foundation. It is adapted from the worklist published in the programme of the Memorial Concert.

PIANO SOLO
Piano Sonatas 1–3 (1955–8)
February Pieces (1959–61) P
Three Winter Potatoes (1961–5) P
Memories of You (1964) UE
Piano Album 1973
Piano Album 1974
Thälmann Variations (1974) EMC
Vietnam Sonata (1976) EMC
We Sing for the Future (1980)

TWO PIANOS
Two Books of Study for Pianists (1958) P
Boolavogue (1981)

CHAMBER MUSIC
Three Pieces for Trumpet and Piano (1955)
String Trios 1 & 2 (1955–6)
Octet 1959 – picc, alto fl, ob, Eb cl, b cl, c bn, vln, cb
First Movement for String Quartet (1961)
The East is Red (1972) – vln, pno
Thälmann Sonata (1974) – vln, perc
Mountains (1977) solo b cl
The Workers' Song (1978) – solo vln

Little Partisan (arr. of Albanian song) (1980) – ob, cl, tenor hn, tbn
Vietnam's Victory (undated) – brass ensemble, also brass band

ORCHESTRAL
Arrangement for Orchestra (1960)
Third Orchestra Piece 1960
Movement for Orchestra (1962) P
Bun No. 1 (1965)
Bun No. 2 (1964) P
Consciously (undated)
Dartmoor (undated)

VOCAL
Voice from Thel's Grave (Blake) (1957) – voice, pno
Ah Thel (Blake) (1963) N – chorus, pno
Soon (Mao) (1971) – unison song
The Proletariat Seeks to Transform the World (1971)
Wild Lilies Bloom Red as Flame (arr. of Chinese revolutionary song) (1972) – sop, chorus, fl, pno; also contralto and instr. ensemble
Chinese Revolutionary Songs *and* Chinese Revolutionary Songs with New Words (1972–3)
Three Bourgeois Songs (Confucian Book of Odes) (1973) EMC – voice, pno
Bethanien Song (1973)
Four Principles on Ireland (1973)
Long Live Chairman Mao (1973)
Revolution is the Main Trend in the World Today (1973)
The Internationale (arr.) (1973) – unison voices, ob, cl, tpt, vc
The Old and the New (1973) – sop, chorus, orch
Il Communismo (1974)
Songs for 'The Exception and the Rule' (Brecht, arr.) (1975) solo voice, chorus, ensemble
Song for the Anti-Imperialists (undated)
Stand Up and Fight (undated)
Sound the Alarm (arr. of Handel) (undated) tenor, brass band
The Croppy Boy (undated)
Watkinson's Thirteen (undated)
There is only one lie, there is only one truth (undated)
Smash the Social Contract (undated)
We Sing for the Future (undated)
Uncatalogued collections of songs for People's Liberation Music and the Progressive Cultural Association

INDETERMINATE INSTRUMENTATION
Autumn '60 (UE) – any instruments

Octet '61 for Jasper Johns (P) – graphic
Solo with Accompaniment (1964) UE – 2
  performers
Material for Harmony Instruments (1964) UE
Volo Solo (1964) P
Treatise (1963–7) P – graphic
Sextet – the Tiger's Mind (1967) P – verbal text
Schooltime Compositions (1968) EMC – verbal,
  graphic, and musical notations
Schooltime Special (1968) EMC – verbal text
The Great Learning (Confucius, trans. Pound)
  (1968–70) EMC
The Great Learning (new trans. by Cardew)
  (1972)

FILM MUSIC
'Strindberg' (1971)
'Sugar' (undated)
'Cold Night' (1974)

DISCOGRAPHY
AMM – AMMusic (1966) Elektra 256 EUK 7256
AMM – Live Electronic Music (1968) (excerpts
  from the Crypt concert – complete as next
  item; this LP also features Musica Elettronica
  Viva) Mainstream MS 5 02
AMM – The Crypt 12 June 1968 (1981) 2 LP
  box set – Matchless MR 5
AMM – Commonwealth Institute 20 April 1967
  (1982) part of compilation album – United
  Dairies 012
The Great Learning Paragraphs 2 & 7 (1971)
  The Scratch Orchestra – Deutsche
  Grammophon 2561 107
Material (1970) in guitar recital by Leo
  Brouwer – Deutsche Grammophon
Four Principles on Ireland and other pieces
  (1974) Cramps CRSLP 6106
Ives – Four Violin Sonatas (1975) Janos
  Negyesy, vln, Cardew, pno – 2 LP box set,
  Thorofon ATHK 136/7
Memorial Concert 16 May 1982 (1985) incl.
  First Movement, Octet '61, Treatise, Great
  Learning, paragraph 1, The Turtledove (from
  3 Bourgeois Songs), The Workers' Song,
  Thälmann Variations, The Croppy Boy,
  Watkinson's Thirteen, Smash the Social
  Contract, There is only one lie, We Sing for
  the Future – Impetus IMP 28204
The release of further recordings is planned,
  including Cardew playing his own piano
  music and the 1984 Great Learning
  performance.

P = Peters Edition
UE = Universal Edition
EMC = Experimental Music Catalogue
N = Novello
All other works are unpublished.

Notes
1 K. Stockhausen, programme note for Carré,
   in K. Wörner, Stockhausen, Life and Work,
   tr. W. Hopkins (Faber, 1973).
2 C. Cardew, 'Report on Stockhausen's Carré',
   The Musical Times, cii, Sept. 1961, pp. 619,
   698.
3 R. de Beer, 'Interview with Stockhausen',
   Key Notes, xvii, 1983/1.
4 C. Cardew, Treatise Handbook (Peters,
   1971).
5 Latimer Press, 1974.
6 Almeida Festival, London, June 1984; the
   performance was split over two
   evenings – paragraphs 1–4 and 5–7 – with
   a total duration of over 9 hours.
7 See Discography.
8 C. Cardew, diary entry for 1 September
   1964, quoted in J. Tilbury, The Music, in
   the programme of the Cardew Memorial
   Concert, Queen Elizabeth Hall, London, 16
   May 1982.
9 C. Cardew, Volo Solo, preface to score (in
   Treatise Handbook).
10 Ibid.
11 Treatise Handbook.
12 Ibid.
13 J. Tilbury, 'Cornelius Cardew', Contact, xxvi,
   Spring 1983.
14 Treatise Handbook.
15 Ibid.
16 Ibid.
17 H. Gilonis, The Ta Hsio of Confucius
   (unpublished translation).
18 In connection with a performance of
   paragraphs 1 and 2 at the Berlin
   Philharmonic Hall in March 1974; the
   essay is included in Stockhausen Serves
   Imperialism.
19 Sleeve note to Deutsche Grammophon
   recording of Paragraphs 2 and 7 – see
   Discography.
20 B. Eno, 'Generating and Organising Variety
   in the Arts', Studio International, Nov./Dec.
   1976.
21 Stockhausen Serves Imperialism.

RICHARD BERNAS

Three Works by Gavin Bryars

*The object of philosophy is to replace concealed
nonsense with revealed nonsense.*

(Ludwig Wittgenstein)

It is rarely an easy or simple matter to discuss the
work of a composer still in his early 40s; still
harder to deal objectively with one with whom you
have frequently collaborated. Rather than pre-
sume a position of defence or attack, I prefer one of
explanation. A number of good articles about
Bryars' work have appeared in *Contact*, so this
essay will forgo lengthy historical background and
concern itself with three recent works: the cantata
Effarene, the opera written in collaboration with
the American director Robert Wilson, *Medea*, and
the String Quartet.

To many listeners, Bryars' work appears
associative, but in calculatedly unpredictable
ways. This is achieved by layering the materials of
a composition so that they are superimposed,
having 'polyphonic' rather than 'harmonic' relationships, and avoiding interpenetration. Each
strata of the musical construction is treated as an
(almost) discrete object, which encourages a yet
more delightful and polyphonic confusion of
associations on the part of the listener.

The most striking precedent for this method is
not found in music, but in the visual arts; in his
conversations with Pierre Cabanne, Marcel
Duchamp spoke about the necessity of avoiding
the merely painterly or retinal approach when
constructing his masterwork *The Large Glass*, in
much the same way as Bryars might avoid the
exclusively sonorous.

> What I put inside was what, will you tell me?
> I was mixing story, anecdote (in the good
> sense of the word), with visual representation,
> while giving less importance to visuality, to
> the visual element, than one generally gives in
> painting. Already I didn't want to be
> preoccupied with visual language . . .
> Everything was becoming conceptual, that is,
> it depended on things other than the retina.

Incidentally, it is worth noting that this position is

parallel to but very different from that of Varèse,
another French-born Modernist whose career in
New York shared Duchamp's pattern of a small
number of works giving rise to a large if belated
sphere of influence.

Naturally, the choice of materials to be
superimposed determines a good deal of the
operation's success, as it would in any composition. For example, though constructed with equal
rigour and along similar lines, the materials used
in Book I of Boulez's *Structures* are, to my ear,
inherently more interesting and satisfying than
those selected by Karel Goeyvaerts in his Sonata for
Two Pianos. Such questions of taste are ultimately
subjective and in a curious way indefensible, so I
will largely ignore them for the remainder of this
article and concentrate on the materials themselves.

Let us consider the elements that make up
Effarene, a forty-minute cantata for soprano,
mezzo-soprano, six percussionists, and four pianists which was premièred in March 1984.

The genesis of this combination needs some
explaining. I asked Bryars for a work which could
use most of the same forces as George Antheil's
'Ballet Mechanique', which would be played at the
same concert. Since Bryars had a large number of
works arranged for various combinations of tuned
percussion and keyboards, this was not as unlikely
a request as it might first appear. He was at the
time occupied with writing some of the music for
Robert Wilson's vast (between eight and fourteen
hours) and as yet not completely realized opera,
Civil wars. The texts of *Effarene* are either from or
associated with Bryars' research on the project,
and the vocal music marked with an asterisk is a
reworking or modification of settings Bryars had
sketched during the opera's many workshops.
They are: a statement by Marie Curie * about the
nature of scientific research, set twice (first con-
templatively, then demonstratively) for soprano; a
poem about the Queen of the Sea by Etel Adnam
* for mezzo-soprano and originally to be sung by
Jessye Norman in Wilson's production; an Ode in
praise of photography by Pope Leo XIII set for

soprano and mezzo; and a text from *20,000 Leagues under the Sea* by Jules Verne about underwater navigation, for mezzo. Except for the Papal Ode, all the texts are in French. The interludes between each vocal setting were adapted from the entractes designed for Bryars' other Wilson collaboration, *Medea*.

The instrumentation is founded on a tuned percussion consort of two marimbas, bass marimba, vibes, glockenspiel, and timpani. All the players double on a wide variety of bells, tuned gongs, cymbals, steel drums, etc. Thus the texture and density of the percussion writing is strikingly different from that of the 'Ballet Mechanique', which emphasizes unpitched instruments, bridges the percussion and piano sounds by means of xylophones, and tries every means – all successful – to make the pianos sound percussive. Inasmuch as a blend of instrumental timbres is intended, *Effarene* recalls the standard Bryars touring ensemble format of two pianos, two tuned percussion (most likely vibraphone and marimba), with a couple of solo instruments. Here this format is writ large, and the increased resource allows for subtle alterations in the voicings of chords within tutti textures as well as allowing the variety expected within a forty-minute composition. The use of tuned percussion ensembles has always been a part of Bryars' teaching – he is Professor of Music at Leicester Polytechnic – and he has a considerable knowledge of their repertory, including their Etudes and Tutors. Many of the figurations used in *Effarene* and for the similarly large percussion consort in *Medea* derive from these sources; percussionists have invariably remarked with approval on the idiomatic nature of these parts.

The last element to consider, after text and orchestration, is that of harmony. Having conducted a reasonably large number of 'postmodern' or 'neo-tonal' scores in the last five years, I've come to the conclusion that a detailed knowledge and experience of jazz harmony is essential for tonal composers working in this decade. Without it, such elementary matters as voice leading, long-range harmonic planning, or the effective (rather than the merely habitual) preparation of cadences seems either overly schematic or clumsy. It has been countered that this clumsiness is a sign of vitality, or at the very least a laudable lack of pretension, but not in my opinion. Bryars' experience as a jazz double-bass player has inevitably influenced his approach to tonal writing and two salient features of his harmonic style can be traced to this background: the use of non-

harmonic passing notes to obscure or enrich simpler chord progressions, and the use of chord substitution at cadential points to redirect the more ordinary processes.

Instances of this approach to harmony, which brings about a kind of scaffolding within the composition which admits an independent – and occasionally unnerving – role of its own as one superimposed strata of composition, are found in the central duet section of *Effarene*. This is a reworking of a chorus from *Civil wars* on the same text, which was composed and rehearsed but never performed. As it started out as a four-part chorus, it seems most conveniently represented that way; here are the harmonies of the first seventeen bars (Ex. 1), the least developed form of the harmonic plan, shown with the harmonic structure of bars 110–22 sketched underneath (Ex. 2). As can be seen, the same harmonies lie at the centre of each of these phrases, and the F major 7 to A flat 6 shift is a focus of much of the duet. Chord substitutions occur throughout, at virtually each repetition of the general pattern, and they are obviously noticed at the start of the second phrase quoted, when the initial shifts between chords with either A or A flat in the bass are glossed over by a sustained period of A flat 2nd inversion. Again at the end of this period, which is the climactic phrase of the duet, expected chords of either A minor plus major 6th or D major 7 are shoved aside by D minor with a major seventh. This is the only appearance of this chord in the duet and the surprise of its appearance is underlined by the voicing of the soprano and mezzo parts, the lower voice momentarily riding over the soprano, and the only appearance of the steel drums. But the steel drums deliver a riff that is jaunty, slightly aggressive and altogether independent of their surroundings (Ex. 3). Within a texture made up of seemingly discrete elements, the momentary fusion of line and harmony, resolutely underlined by contradictory elements of the orchestration (that is to say, the entry of the steel drums) makes a strong and disconcertingly elegant impression.

In this duet, the orchestration of the instrumental parts is for the most part concerned with varied chord voicings between pianos and marimbas; the four pianos are spread over a wide range, but each plays a compactly voiced chord; contrarywise, the spacing of the three marimbas' chords are wider and their sonority is maintained by soft-stick tremolos. When two marimbas play in unison, it is to pick out a sequence of notes from the middle of the overall harmonic texture and to accentuate it as a form of counter-melody to the

Example 1

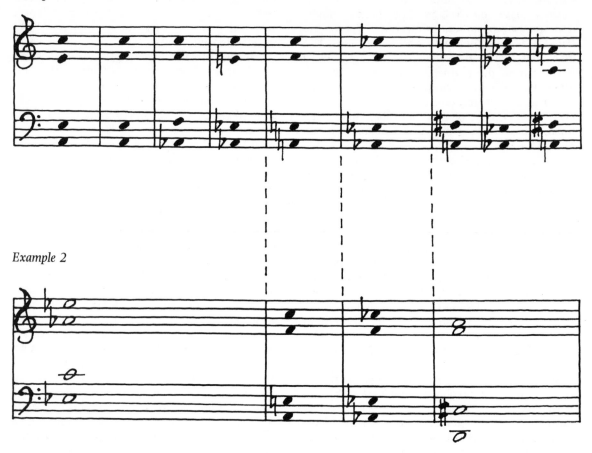

Example 2

Example 3

Soprano and Mezzo

steel drums

voice parts. The percussion bass line is exchanged between bass marimba and timpani, and as a harmonic punctuation each F major 7 first inversion chord is reinforced by tightly spaced vibraphone and glockenspiel entries. Against repeated, shorter piano patterns, the vocal lines proceed in long periods of four to seven bars. They move smoothly and conjunctly, a very French texture that sounds like early Fauré and which forms an ironic balance to the Latin dignity and reserve of the Papal text.

The superimposition of styles mentioned above when describing the use of steel drums during the duet again comes to the fore at the end of *Effarene,* a section Bryars composed specifically for the work. Rather than a reworking of *Civil wars* related material, it is the setting of a text that might have been used in the opera; since a good deal of the action takes place under the sea, Bryars uses Jules Verne's catalogue of underwater geographical places of interest. The mezzo-soprano sings this in a leisurely, Berlioz-style recitative, in free, floating time and accompanied by measured, 'graceful' arpeggios played by the pianos. At the same time, the bass marimba delivers a stealthy walking-bass, rhythmically steady and jazzy in profile, reinforced by lightly brushed cymbal strokes and again remarkably independent of its surroundings. The effect of the two combined is easily analysed (no interpenetration at all – end of question) but difficult to describe. Imagine someone giving a very proper recital of mélodies at home, and then introduce the neighbours, a couple of houses down the block, having a loud reggae party of which only the thudding bass and the odd whispy sizzle leak through the cosy double glazing.

An application of similar resources in a parallel set of circumstances can be observed in the duet between Medea and Aegeus that opens Act III of Bryars' opera. This was the last music written for *Medea,* composed only six or seven weeks before the première in October 1984. The text was first set in 1982, and was conceived specifically for an earlier production of the opera, at La Fenice, Venice, which was cancelled because of technical problems. For this staging, both the roles of Medea and Aegeus were to be played by black singers, as they had been in Robert Wilson's earliest workshop productions of Euripides' play. In the context of the play, these two characters are old and trusted friends and the scene is a relatively relaxed conversation between them amidst Medea's highly strung confrontations with Jason. Bryars conceived it in a loose jazz style, rather like the big band scores of Ellington or Evans. But the 1984 production of *Medea* at the Opéra de Lyon was completely recast, so Medea was sung by an Australian soprano (Yvonne Kenney) and Aegeus by a French baritone (Pierre Yves le Magat). Their conversation in bebop and scat phrases was more than ironic – it proved dramatically incredible. In addition, the management of the theatre persuaded Wilson and Bryars to translate all the passages of Euripides' text which Wilson had originally planned (and Bryars set) in English into French, which made the jazz style sit even less well on the scene as a whole. The opening of Act III occurs directly after the interval; it was a crucial place in the sequence of the opera, and something had to be done.

In order to produce the new music at short notice, Bryars took over the harmonic plan of the *Effarene* duet I have described above, over which he composed the vocal lines using the same rhythmic stresses for the phrases to be sung in Greek as had existed in the Venice version (but obviously recomposing the pitches) and setting the new French translation from scratch. Now advocates of a Gesamtkunstwerk theory of art will inevitably squirm at such tactics, but these processes are not dissimilar to those employed by composers in the early nineteenth century when forced into similar operatic circumstances. The music that accompanies part of the finale of Act I of *The Barber of Seville* also serves to underline Otello's increasing jealousy in his duet with Desdemona in Rossini's version of that play. This was not considered an error, but rather a manifestation of a neo-classical concept of opera, in which the text has the central role of generating emotion, and the music allows it to do so. The orchestral accompaniment was then composed in relation to the vocal lines and harmony. As in his other works, Bryars' orchestral forces are (slightly) unusual in *Medea*: as well as the six percussion already mentioned when considering *Effarene*, much use is made of divisi strings, yet there are no violins. (Curious that, about 150 years after the last opera to dispense altogether with violins, Méhul's *Uthal*, both Bryars and Philip Glass should decide on this tactic at roughly the same time.) The rest of the orchestra is more usual, though the absence of oboes and trumpets, and the addition of two saxophones, must be noted.

Possibly because of the pressure to produce a radically different rendering of the text, or possibly out of the pleasure of being in continuous contact with the (extremely helpful) singers and of having the considerable resources of an opera house at his disposal, this scene must be accounted one of the most successful in the opera. The use of the voices is very free and flexible (see Ex. 4); the orchestral lines are closely integrated with the vocal parts, remarking on them as well as accompanying. Some anomaly exists inasmuch as the music is extremely Romantic when compared to the severe scenes preceding it, but Bryars defuses this tendency at the end of the duet by citing, in a two-bar 'window', the walking-bass bebop style of the Venice version, a transition that, without the explanations I've given, strikes listeners as inexplicable, unpredictable, and disconcerting, since it fits on a purely historical rather than aesthetic level.

The writing found in the rest of the opera can be roughly classified into two categories; 'before and after winter 1982'. For six weeks during this period, Robert Wilson rehearsed in workshop conditions the first half of the opera. The timings between scenes, the pacing of entrances and exits, the fine details of the vocal lines, were all refined and tested at New York City College, with many of the intended original (Venetian) cast and in conditions like that of a piano/stage rehearsal at a fully professional opera house. This is a costly business, but it is the usual way Wilson works with his collaborators; the gestation of *Einstein on the Beach* took place in such workshops, spread over a three-year period. Having participated in these

weeks and seen the changes in the composer's attitude towards the stage that this continual but unpressured contact brought about, I cannot help regretting that such opportunities are not made a precondition of any contemporary operatic creation.

A striking example of 'before winter 1982' is the scene that closes Act II, and so precedes the Medea/Aegus duet. This is the first of three duets between Medea and Jason, which sums up the action so far and reinforces the tensions that have built up in Euripides' text. The core of the scene is a percussion toccata in hard-driving, repetitive 'Nexus' style, over which the protagonists declaim in tightly moving vocal patterns. Sections of the text which Wilson designed to be spoken rather than sung are treated as inserts, with completely static, revolving figuration in the percussion, played at a notably slower tempo. Whenever the main thrust of the (sung) argument resumes, the orchestration is enriched and elaborated, so that very gradually, over fifteen minutes, the entire orchestra is playing for the first time in the Act. Another set of inserts are the declamatory interruptions of the chorus, observing the debate and commenting on it in the manner of judges at a tribunal. The overall effect is one of a long line, gradually growing thicker and more dense without resolving in any definite way, but rather

Example 4

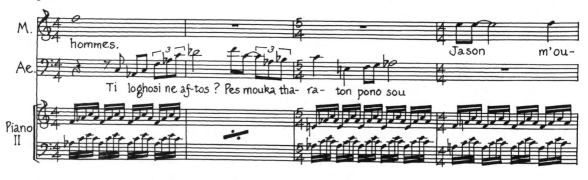

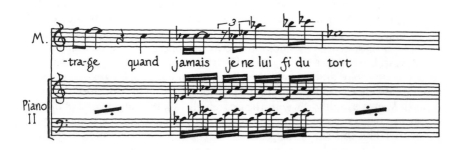

coming to rest on the music given to Medea after Jason leaves; it is schematic writing of considerable invention and resource, which makes a strong impression on the audience because of the long-range energy which it conveys.

The music written 'after winter 1982' is not vastly different in style or suitability for the stage, but it is more subtly written for both voices and orchestra. There is a flexibility in it that critics of the 40s and 50s used to term 'plastic' before that word became associated solely with mass production, and it seems to me obviously the result of Bryars' encounter with his singers, on stage, in the workshop period. It is also more closely aligned to the overall conception of the stage pictures Wilson had invented for *Medea*. The action of the play takes place outside Medea's house. Wilson intensified the impact of each of the succeeding Acts by bringing the house closer to the audience, making it occupy more and more of the stage: in Act I we see the house with four classical columns in front of it; by Act IV the house is so large that the doorway dwarfs the singers and obscures the sky, with only one column, about five feet across, set in the middle of the stage, threatening the spectators. When such a zoom process is controlled gradually over three hours, the effect is felt rather than perceived, and the claustrophobia projected by the stage was palpable.

Bryars' response to this disciplined simplicity was to invent musical devices that would 'read' in the theatre, with a boldness of style and a fearlessness about courting the obvious which compliments and enhances the larger manoeuvres of the stage. The best example of this is in the penultimate scene, the last of Medea and Jason's confrontations. A restless and obsessive dotted quaver plus semiquaver pulse accompanies Jason's lines throughout the opening, a variant of the classic anapaestic rhythm of Verdi's death scenes. When Medea enters, flying down from the top of the proscenium on a golden chariot drawn by two serpents, the rhythm that dominates her music is the same figure, played twice as long. The figures overlap, and despite the spectacular nature of the stage picture, the audience perceives the link between them. In this respect the music fulfils one of the major requirements of an operatic score, that of being completely intelligible to the audience in the theatre.

Unfortunately, one of the finest purely musical passages of the score never got as far as the première. One of the drawbacks of Wilson's brilliant stage designs was the large amount of wing space they took up in the Lyon Opera, a theatre built during the 1830s to accommodate flat painted scenery. This more than doubled the time that was allocated for some of the scene changes, necessitating additional internal repeats in music originally designed to link scenes together in a rather more direct, less bombastic way. The difficulties in quickly shifting these large constructions also led to the wholesale deletion of one of Wilson's most interesting scenes, a representation of the death of Creon's daughter, all on fire, throwing herself off a cliff into the sea. This was to be portrayed by a half-size puppet far upstage on an enormous and very solid looking cliff face, and sung by a wordless soprano, often staying for bars on end well above the stave, positioned in the orchestra pit. Bryars had conceived this scene as a set of harmonic variations based around a central pedal A, always repeated somewhere in the orchestra. The soloistic and harmonic shifts of this passage are the epitome of Bryars' rigorous avoidance of the obvious, despite the use of familiar materials. This was clearly represented even by the visual aspect of the score, as the repeated As are only played by transposing instruments or C clef instruments, and so superficially look like different notes while sounding always the same pitch; an ironic comment enjoyed, in this case, only by the conductor of the performance. The scene is Bryars' strongest orchestral work to date, and it is a pity that it has yet to be played in public.

Few theatre works are perfect, there are invariably too many exigencies involved. But having observed the gestation of this opera over a period of more than four years, it seems to me that composers who embark on this form need as much time and opportunity to revise and adjust their work as can possibly be given, and then more time to finely tune it. At a time when the concept of opera is gaining renewed credibility as a contemporary form, thanks in some large part to the efforts of Wilson himself, the idea of professional or at least semi-professional workshop periods for a duration longer than the rehearsal periods most festival productions of existing works enjoy might seem unrealistic. But one director can do it, so others who are interested must simply work towards the ideal of similar conditions for the good of their own and their collaborators' work. Bryars is now actively involved in discussions for two more works with other directors and producers, both a full-scale and a chamber opera. It will be much to his credit if he can succeed in creating circumstances which will enable him to fulfil these projects at the same high standard that he realized with Wilson – something Philip Glass, another

Wilson collaborator, has not always succeeded in achieving.

The avoidance of the obvious despite obvious means is an important concern of Bryars' recent String Quartet, which has been recorded by the Arditti Quartet for ECM Records. As an etude in the deflation of expectations it asks a major question – does good writing always mean idiomatic writing? – and answers with a deeply felt 'perhaps not'.

The alternation between good, idiomatic string writing, so obvious to most listeners that it seems unnecessary to quote an example of it here, and long sections based on figurations which can most simply be summarized as pianistic, occurs in rigorous alternation throughout the Quartet. In every case, I find the passages that sit clumsily on the medium to be more interesting, not because they 'sound wrong' but because they ask questions which ought to be posed. These questions are answered and in some respect (unsatisfactorily) resolved by more conventional textures, but never with sufficient thoroughness to conclude the discussion.

An example of what can be summarized by a pianistic texture is given in Example 5, which has a Thalberg-like solidity. It is not difficult to see the right hand playing the violin arpeggios and handling their hairpin crescendo and diminuendo chords with a tremolo, while the left neatly takes care of the viola and cello octaves. This format is repeated enough times to become predictable, when glissandi are introduced to the 'left hand', reminding the listener that means other than a keyboard are being employed. The section lasts for some 40 bars, with an increasing use of glissandi in the viola and cello parts. Questions as to what is the best vehicle for these sounds become more insistent, until the tensions are neutralized by a five-bar phrase of Ravelian texture, in which the quartet delivers, with delicately overlapping arpeggiations, an harmonic sequence that would not be out of place in a Gounod opera: C major; C augmented triad; F major with a flattened 6th; C major. This plagal cadence with added perfume paves the way for the central and most perplexing section of the Quartet. Up to this point, the majority of the melodic material used has been developed from arpeggiations of chord sequences. The cadence cited above and a short transitional passage introduce a series of scales, from middle C to the octave above, played at first by both violins. Each of the scales is inflected with different accidentals, starting with a flattened second; then

a flattened fifth; flattened second and fifth; flattened second and sixth; and so on. Bryars reviews virtually all of the scales expounded by Busoni in his famous passage about Infinite Harmony and the future of tonality from the *Sketch for a New Esthetic of Music*:

> I have made an attempt to exhaust the possibilities of the arrangement of degrees within a seven-tone scale; and succeeded, by raising and lowering the intervals, in establishing one hundred and thirteen different scales . . . There is a significant difference between the sound of the scale C–D flat–E flat–F flat–G flat–A flat–B flat–C when C is taken as tonic, and the scale of D flat major. By giving the customary C major triad as a fundamental harmony, a novel harmonic sensation is obtained. But now listen to this same scale supported alternatively by the A minor, E flat major, and C major triads, and you cannot avoid a feeling of delightful surprise at the strangely unfamiliar euphony.

The permutation of these scales, winding slowly up and down over a fairly static ground of (for the most part) pedal Cs and harmonized in blissfully non-functional ways, creates the most bewildering and hypnotic experience in Bryars' recent music. The question of non-idiomatic, pianistic writing again occurs, especially as Bryars is here presenting the philosophical speculations of a famous composer-pianist, but the length of the passage and its even flow soon concentrate the ear on the notes and not their source. In the recorded version, each of the scales Bryars selects is played once; at the first (Vienna) performance all these passages were repeated, and at a subsequent (London) performance a selection of some scales were repeated while others were not. Having read through the score, I found the recorded version the least successful; since proportions of musical paragraphs are important to a composer's thought, the shortening of this section makes it superficially sound more like an extended transition section between the less severe material on either side of it than a statement of central importance to the Quartet. Without the repeats, the Quartet strikes an uneasy balance, especially as the succeeding music is unabashedly lyrical, with demonstratively violinistic figurations supporting a long viola melody. This music is presented in the key of B major, onto which the repeated C to C scales appear to sink. In the passage

Example 5

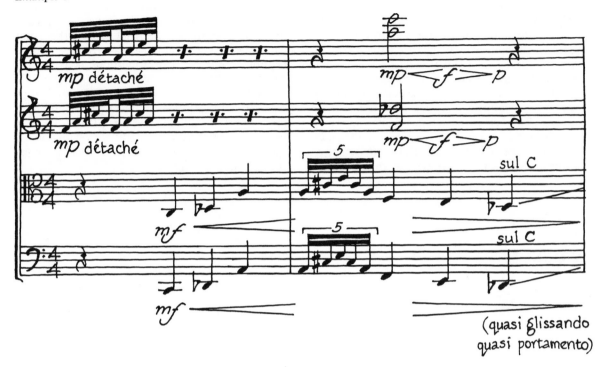

(quasi glissando
quasi portamento)

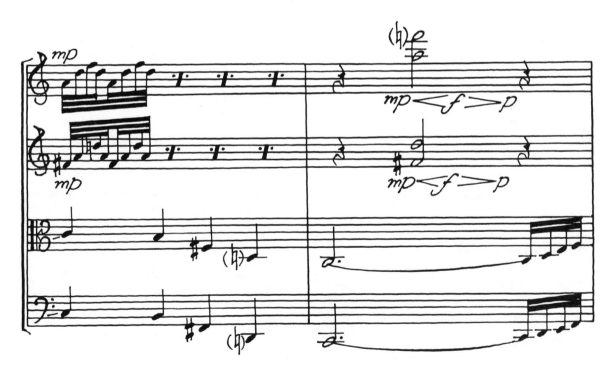

41

that follows the viola melody, each of the string instruments in turn tunes down to lower pitches, so, for example, the first violin tunes down the E and A strings to D sharp and G sharp. After this operation is completed, in a passage that creates a (yet another) rather disturbing effect in performance though not on disc, each member of the quartet in turn plays an ascending scale or sequence of natural harmonics on the retuned strings. This elegant statement, bewilderingly arrived at, is an acoustic answer to the philosophical ramblings of Busoni's premise, to which it forms a brief but important ballast. Or it might be heard as an example of Duchamp's 'anecdote (in the good sense of the word)'.

Such speculative music leaves an uneasy impression on the listener that expects the usual certitudes of neo-tonal music from Bryars. It must be noted that his works without texts are in general more elliptical and ambiguous than, for example *Effarene*, and that work is contradictory enough. Is his attitude completely new, and how far is it an extension of older precedents? 'There is no new or old. Only known and not yet known. Of these, it seems to me the known still forms by far the smaller part.' (Busoni.)

WORKLIST

compiled by Andrew Thomson, July 1986

Works marked with an asterisk are available for hire or purchase from:
> Mnemonic Ltd,
> Andrew Thomson,
> 48 Etta Street,
> Deptford,
> London SE8 5NT
> telephone 01 692 0032

Works without the asterisk are not available for public performance.

Gavin Bryars is exclusively managed and represented by:
> Erica Bolton & Jane Quinn Ltd
> 130 Hammersmith Grove,
> London W6 7HB
> telephone 01 846 9337/01 748 9183

Pre-mature pieces

1965–6
Catalogue   pno(s) with or without tape (ms. lost)

1966
For a Birthday   pno (ms. lost)
Hoyu Spoke No Words   tpt, sax, guitar, cb, drums (ms. John Cage)
Visions   ensemble of bass instruments and perc

1967
16 Continuous Fragments for 2 Guitars   (ms. Derek Bailey)
Three No. 7   2 pnos, 6 hands, tape

1968
3 solos for piano   (ms. lost)
From 3 Upwards   theatre piece (two parts used for renamed piece: *In order that you may set the whole world an example in discretion I will tell you no more about it*   Verbal Anthology, Experimental Music Catalogue (EMC)
Three No. 5   tape piece (lost)
Eggeling Music   indeterminate (ms. lost)
Notice the Dulcet Quality, the Tonal Translucency of the Majestic Waltz   1, 2, or 3 pnos

1969
Portsmouth   indeterminate, verbal piece
St. Augustine   indeterminate, verbal piece

Mature pieces

1968
*Mr. Sunshine   any number of keybds, including one prepared pno. 1st perf: Kingston College of Art, 13 Dec. 1968 (John Tilbury, hpschd; G.B., pno; tapes); BBC broadcast (*sic*!) 5 Sept. 1970 (John Tilbury, org; Howard Skempton, org pedals; stereo tapes); (also published in EMC Keyboard Anthology, and separately).
*Made in Hong Kong   indeterminate, verbal piece. 1st perf: Central School of Art, Feb. 1969 (G.B. and students); (also published in EMC Verbal Anthology).
The Music-Lover's Portfolio   (tape and live sounds). Recorded: London, 29 Aug. 1968, (Derek Bailey, guitar; G.B., tape).

1969
*Marvellous Aphorisms are scattered richly throughout these pages   solo theatre piece. 1st perf: Students' Union, University College, Cardiff, 6 Nov. 1969 (G.B.); (also published in EMC Verbal & Visual Anthologies).
A Must for all Sibelians   Tape piece. 1st perf: Helsinki, 1970, during Systems Art exhibition

Some of the interesting things you'll see on a long-distance flight   tape and live sounds
Private Music   1st perf: Reardon-Smith Hall, Cardiff, 1969; (also published in EMC Verbal Anthology).
The Sinking of the Titanic   indeterminate (possible materials include: 2 stereo tapes, 4-part string ensemble, perc (woodblocks and alarm clock), 2 low brass, (preferably tba & hn), brass quintet, 1 cassette tape of speech, pno or harmonium, 35 mm slides, visible sound effects, music box); 1st perf: Queen Elizabeth Hall, London, 1972 (*Music Now Ensemble*, directed by G.B.); (partial score in *Soundings*, 9 (1975)).
Golders (as) Green by Eps(ups)om(n) Downs (also published in EMC Visual Anthology).

1970
Pre-Medieval Metrics   unspecified ensemble. BBC 2 'Art & Technology' series, Nov. 1970; (also published in EMC Rhythmic Anthology).
The Harp that once through Tara's Halls   never performed – imperfectly realized Waterloo Station summer 1970; (also published in EMC Verbal Anthology).
Serenely Beaming and Leaning on a Five-Barred Gate   1st perf: Portsmouth College of Art, 14 Jan. 1970 (John Tilbury, Liz Mason, Gary Rickard); simultaneous performance of *Marvellous Aphorisms . . .* by G.B.; (also published in EMC Verbal Anthology).
Ouse   theatre piece for 2 singers. 1st perf: Black Swan, York, 30 Nov. 1984 (*Soundpool* series: Nick Williams, Dave King, Tim Brooks); (also published in EMC Visual Anthology).
The Ride Cymbal and the Band that caused the Fire in the Sycamore Trees   1 or 2 prepared pnos. 1st perf: Purcell Room, 9 Oct. 1970 (John Tilbury, prepared pno; G.B., tapes); version with ensemble: Palais des Beaux-Arts, Brussels, Feb. 1973 (G.B. & Christopher Hobbs, prepared pnos; string ensemble, conductor John White); (also published in EMC Keyboard Anthology, reprinted in *Soundings*, 9 (1975)).
To gain the affections of Miss Dwyer even for one short minute would benefit me no end   imperfect private perf, Portsmouth College of Art, Nov. 1970; (also published in EMC Visual Anthology).
A Game of Football   (published in EMC Visual Anthology).

1971
1, 2, 1-2-3-4   ensemble. Dedicated to John White; 1st perf: Bluecoat Hall, Liverpool (*Music Now Ensemble*: Howard Skempton, G.B., Christopher Hobbs, Michael Parsons, Hugh Shrapnel, Sandra Hill, Alec Hill); (also published in EMC Verbal Anthology).
The Chair of BlaBlaBla   (composed but never realized).

The Squirrel and the Ricketty-Racketty Bridge   guitars. Commissioned by Derek Bailey; 1st perf: Queen Elizabeth Hall, Dec. 1972 (Derek Bailey, John Tilbury); (also published in EMC Rhythmic Anthology).
Jesus' Blood Never Failed Me Yet   tape and ensemble. 1st perf: Queen Elizabeth Hall, Dec. 1972; Recording used for film by Steve Dwoskin, 1971; (also published by EMC).

1972
The Heat of the Beat   not yet performed (also published in EMC Verbal Anthology).
A Place in the Country   not yet performed (also published in EMC Visual Anthology).
Far Away and Dimly Pealing   imperfect (i.e. incomplete) perf only (also published in EMC Verbal Anthology).

1975
Long-Player   up to 3 strings and pno. 1st perf: *George W. Welch*, University of Keele, 16 Nov. 1983; (also published in EMC String Supplement).
Ponukelian Melody (10')   i) original version: vc, tba, harmonium, tubular bells; 1st perf: Lucy Milton Gallery, 15 May 1975; later issued on *Audio Arts* cassette, Vol. 3 No. 2   ii) 'tour' version: bells, mar, timp, vc, reed org (or casio), pno, cb; 1st perf: Midland Institute, Birmingham, 5 Nov. 1981   iii) arr. Andrew Thomson: bells, mar, tba, string quartet, pno; 1st perf: *George W. Welch*, BMIC, 21 June 1984   iv) 2 pno version; 1st perf Stedelijk Museum, Amsterdam, 26 Jan. 1980 (G.B. and John White).

1976
White to Play (and win)   perc trio. 1st perf: Palais des Beaux-Arts, Brussels, 1 Feb. 1976 (John White, G.B., Christopher Hobbs).
Tra-la-la-lira-lira-lay   (formerly entitled *Detective Fiction and Related Subjects*)   1st perf: ICC Antwerp, 15 May 1976 (John White, tba; G.B., vc; Chris Hobbs, reed org; Angela Bryars, slides/tapes).

1977
Irma   opera, realization of Tom Phillips' work. No live perf.
The Perfect Crime   2 pnos, tape, perc, opt slides. 1st perf: Free University of Brussels, 1 Apr. 1977 (G.B., pno; Stuart Marshall, perc; Chris Hobbs, pno; Angela Bryars, slides).
First Suite from 'Irma'   2 pnos 1st perf: Palais des Beaux-Arts, Brussels, 2 Apr. 1977 (Christopher Hobbs & G.B.).
White's SS (18')   i) version for 2 pnos: 1st perf: Centrum Bellevue, Amsterdam (Holland Festival), 10 June 1977 (G.B. and John White)   ii) 2 pnos 4 hands, 3 players at one mar, opt tba: 1st perf: Chapelle de la Sorbonne, Paris (Festival d'Automne), 16 Nov. 1979.
R+7   perc duo. 1st perf: Centrum 't Hoogt,

Utrecht (Holland Festival), 12 June 1977 (G.B. & Christopher Hobbs).
Poggioli in Zaleski's Gazebo pno, tba, tuned perc. 1st perf: Air Gallery, London, 1 Nov. 1977 (Amanda Hurton, vibes; Arthur Soothill, xylophone; John White, tba; G.B., pno; Dave Smith, bells).
Out of Zaleski's Gazebo (12'30") 2 pnos, 6 or 8 hands. 1st perf: University of Louvain, Belgium, 8 Dec. 1977 (G.B., Christopher Hobbs, John White).

1978

Danse Dieppoise i) hn, tba, pno, vibes. 1st perf: Stedelijk Museum, Amsterdam, 15 Apr. 1978 (G.B., Ben Mason, John White, Dave Smith) ii) hn, tbn, fl, cl, hpschd.
My First Homage (17'30") i) 2 pnos. 1st perf: Kitchen, New York, 10 Nov. 1978 (G.B. & Dave Smith); (used for the play *The Golden Windows* by Robert Wilson) ii) 2 pnos + solo vibes, *or* 1 vibes 4 hands, *or* 2 vibes, *or* 2 vibes (2nd part simple) + opt cb &/or tba. 1st perf: Chapelle de la Sorbonne, Paris (Festival d'Automne), 16 Nov. 1979 iii) 'tour version'. 2 sax, 2 vibes, pno, tba, cb, perc (bells & sizzle cymbal) 1st perf: Midland Institute, Birmingham, 5 Nov. 1981.
2nd Suite from 'Irma' pno & string orch. Not yet performed – planned performance in Venice 1978.

1979

Ramsey's Lamp (8') 2 pnos, 6 hands. 1st perf: ICA London, 4 Feb. 1979 (G.B., Dave Smith, John White).
Epsom Downs perc quartet. 1st perf: School of Performing Arts, Scraptoft, Leicester, 20 June 1979 (with dance).
Sforzesco Sforzando 4 pnos. 1st perf: Castello Sforzesca, Milan, 23 June 1979 (Danilo Lorenzi, Gisella Belgeri, Antonio Ballista, G.B., pnos; theatre event organized by CRT).
Epsom Downs mark 2 perc duo. Not yet performed (intended for CRT event Castello Sforzesca, Milan, 23 June 1979, but due to scale of room, improvisation by John White, bells; & G.B., vibes, substituted).
The Cross-Channel Ferry (13') Elastic scoring. Ensemble comprises: i) pno ii) 2 mars; *or* 1 mar & 1 bass mar; *or* 1 mar & 1 vibes; *or* 1 mar iii) vla; &/or vln; &/or treble viol; opt cl; &/or 2nd vln iv) v; &/or b cl; &/or tba or cb; opt steel drums & shakers (maracas, chocolo). 1st perf: Chapelle de la Sorbonne, Paris (Festival d'Automne), 16 Nov. 1979.

1980

The Vespertine Park (12') 1 or 2 pnos; 2 vibes *or* 1 vibes & 1 mar; mar *or* b mar/bells; opt steel drums/sizzle cymbal. 1st perf: Musée d'Art Moderne, Paris (Paris Biennale), 25 Oct. 1980.
The English Mail-Coach (4'30") perc quartet (2 vibes 8 hands/roto-toms). 1st perf: Air Gallery, London, 23 April 1980.

After Mendelssohn pno duet. 1st perf: Musée d'Art Moderne, Paris, 26 Oct. 1980 (John White & G.B.).
Sidescraper pno duet. Commissioned by *Dancework*, choreography and solo dancer Christine Juffs; 1st perf: Sept. 1980 (G.B. & John White).
Hi-Tremolo (12') vibes, mar (or vibes), 2 pnos. 1st perf: Musée d'Art Moderne, Paris (Paris Biennale), 26 Oct. 1980.

1981

Sixteen tape. Commissioned by *Dancework*, choreography Christine Juffs.
Prologomenon to 'Medea' (12') cl, b cl, mar, b mar, vc, cb, 2 casios, timps. 1st perf: Midland Institute, Birmingham, 5 Nov. 1981.

1982(–4)

Medea (3 hr 45') opera. Libretto after Euripides; direction and design: Robert Wilson; dedication: Richard Bernas. 1st perf: Opéra de Lyon, France, 23 Oct. 1984 (conductor Richard Bernas), ran for 6 nights then moved to Théâtre des Champs-Elysées, Paris for a further 5 nights; (Co-production: Opéra de Lyon, Opéra de Paris, Festival d'Automne). Partial staged run-through (in dress, pno accomp): City College, New York, Mar. 1982 (conductor Richard Bernas); the Prologue, Act 1 (complete), Act 2 (complete), Act 4C, and Act 5C were performed on this occasion.

1983

Grey Windows tape (for dance). 1st perf: Phoenix Theatre Leicester, Apr. 1983 Choreography; Tony Thatcher; Film by David Robinson.
Three Studies on Medea (35') 2 pnos, mar, 2 vibes, bells, cymbal (sizzle), cl, tenor hn, strings. 1st perf: Secession Hall, Vienna, 22 May 1983 (conductor Richard Bernas).
Allegrasco (12'30") sop sax (or cl) and pno. Commissioned by Jan Steele with funds made available by West Midlands Arts; 1st perf: (sax version) Leicester University, 7 Dec 1983 (Jan Steele, Janet Sherbourne).
Civil wars opera (incomplete). Collaboration with Robert Wilson, originally scheduled for performance at the Los Angeles Olympics, but unperformed to date. Some sections of the music exist in completed form, as follows:
i) *Ars Photographica* SATB chorus, harmonium, pno. Text: Pope Leo XIII. Rehearsed, but not recorded, in July 1983, in Baden-Baden. Section II of this work (which is in 3 sections), subsequently became the Latin duet in *Effarene* (see below).
ii) *2B* perc ensemble. 3 pieces of contrasting character. No. 2 was re-notated (it was originally in free tempo) to become the accomp to the solo hn in *Viennese Dance No. 1 (M.H.)* (see below); No. 3 subsequently formed the basis for the final section of *Les Fiancailles* (see below); recorded Baden-Baden, Südwestfunk, Mar. 1983.

iii) Arias for: Marie Curie, The Queen of the Sea, Captain Nemo, The Japanese Bride (in Japanese and French). Workshop rehearsals and performance at 'La Sainte Baume' Monastery, near Marseille, France, Feb. 1984 (sections of this workshop were filmed by Howard Brookner for BBC 2's *Arena* documentary about Robert Wilson).
Les Fiancailles (17' 30") 2 pnos 8 hands, string quintet (2, 1, 1, 1) opt 2 vibes & sizzle cymbal. 1st perf: Secession Hall, Vienna, 22 May 1983 (conductor Richard Bernas).

1984
Effarene (40') sop, mezzo-sop, 4 (or 2) pnos, 6 perc, text: Marie Curie, Etel Adnam, Pope Leo XIII, Jules Verne; 1st perf: St John's, Smith Square, London (Macnaghten Concert) 23 Mar. 1984, (conductor Richard Bernas).
Hymne a la Rrose (6') French 'village' band (fanfare). Commissioned for unveiling of statue of Rrose Selavy in Rouen.

1984–5
Eglisak (22'40") i) 2 pnos, 2 vlns, perc, 1st perf: Rote Fabrik, Zurich, 28 Apr. 1985 ii) chamber orch, 1st perf: Conservatoire de Strasbourg, 10 Oct. 1985.

1985
Homage to Vivier (10') fl, cl, vibes, pno. 1st perf: Almeida Theatre, London, 1 July 1985 *(Lontano)*.
String Quartet No. 1 ('Between the National and the Bristol') (23') Dedicated to Hazel Davies (1931–85); commissioned by the Vienna Festival, for the Arditti Quartet; 1st perf: Messe Palatz, Vienna, 8 Oct. 1985 (Arditti Quartet).
Viennese Dance No. 1 (M.H.) (20') hn (+ opt 2nd hn), string trio *or* string quartet, 6 perc.

1985–6
Pico's Flight (25') sop voice and orch (2 fl, picc, 2 ob (CA), 2 cl (b cl), bn, cbn, 3 hn, 2 tpt, 2 tbn, pno, 2 perc, timp, strings (5, 5, 5, 3)). Text: after Pico della Mirandola; commissioned by the Royal Holloway College, Egham, for its centenary; 1st perf: Royal Holloway College, 25 Feb. 1986.

1986
Sub Rosa ensemble. Commissioned by Sub Rosa; 1st perf: Ghent (Festival of Flanders), 10 Nov. 1986.
Doctor Ox's Experiment (Capitro VI) sop and ensemble. Text after Jules Verne, in Esperanto; commissioned by Festival of Flanders; 1st perf: Ghent (Festival of Flanders), 10 Nov. 1986.

Miscellaneous

1966–74 Music for films by Franco Brocani, Steve Dwoskin, Jean Genet.
Since 1984 worked in jazz group *Nardis* (G.B., cb; Conrad Cork, alto sax; occasionally John Runcie, drums).

1986 Improvisation with Pascal Pongy (hn) and Charles Fulbrook (perc) for record on ECM New Series (1323). This appears twice on the disc (as *Prologue* and *Epilogue*).

Writings and Articles

Art & Artists, Oct. 1972: review of reprint of La Monte Young and Jackson Maclow: *An anthology*
Music & Musicians, Dec. 1972: review of concerts Since 1975: regular reviews for *British Book News*
by *Taj Mahal Travellers* and *Tele Topa* at ICES Festival, London
EMC Anthology: Portsmouth Sinfonia, Robin Mortimore, and James Lampard
Studio International, Nov./Dec. 1976: *Berners, Rousseau, Satie; Notes on Marcel Duchamp's Music;* (with Fred Orton) interviews with *Tom Phillips, Morton Feldman*
Studio International, Apr. 1977: *Duchamp in France* (galley proofs ready when the magazine went bankrupt)
1978: *Portrait of Lord Berners* sleeve notes for Unicorn Records (RHS 355)
1979: *Lord Berners* exhibition catalogue, Autunno Musicale, Como, Italy
July 1982: *Erato au service du crime* (Organographes du Cymbalum Pataphysicum)
Contact, xxv, Autumn 1982: *Satie and the British Contact,* xxvi, Spring 1983: *Vexations and its performers*
Albanian Summer by Dave Smith sleeve notes for record *(Practical 2)* of Smith's piece
29 Oct. 1985: *John White and Friends* programme notes for concert given at St John's, Smith Square (New Macnaghten).
Work in progress: book on Lord Berners (Faber, projected date of publication, 1988).
Bryars has also lectured widely in Great Britain and America. He is currently Professor of Music at the School of Performing Arts, Leicester Polytechnic

Discography

1971 (Incus 2) *The Squirrel and the Ricketty-Racketty Bridge* (Derek Bailey)
1975 (Obscure 1; Edition EG EGED 21) *The Sinking of the Titanic; Jesus' Blood Never Failed Me Yet* (ensembles directed by G.B.)
(Obscure 2) *1, 2, 1-2-3-4* (ensemble directed by G.B.)
1976 (Obscure 8; Edition EG EGED 28) *The Squirrel and the Ricketty-Racketty Bridge* (G.B., Bailey, Fred Frith, Brian Eno)
1977 (Obscure 9; Edition EGED 29) *Irma*, an opera, with Tom Phillips and Fred Orton
(Audio Arts Vol. 3 No. 2) *Ponukelian Melody* (with White and Hobbs)
1980 (Pipe 2) *After Mendelssohn* (G.B. & John White)

(Crepuscule TW1 007) *White's SS*
1981 (Crepuscule TW1 027) 'Hommages'
containing *My First Homage; The English Mail-Coach; The Vespertine Park; Hi-Tremolo*
1986 (ECM New Series 1323) 'Three Viennese
Dancers' containing *Prologue; String Quartet*
No. 1, 1st Viennese Dance; Epilogue
(Sub Rosa 3) *Sub Rosa* (with music by John
Hassell, Harold Budd, and some Gregorian chant)

My thanks to Gavin Bryars for his co-operation
during the production of this list.

Piano Pieces

This portfolio of miniature piano pieces, mostly specially composed and all published for the first time, does not pretend or even aim to give a comprehensive survey of compositional activity in this country. Firstly, the sheer variety of that achievement would have necessitated a far larger selection (for reasons of space alone impossible in this publication) to have even begun to be fully representative. Secondly, and more simply, there were limits to the number of composers we knew well enough to ask, persuade, blackmail, and so on. Although, undeniably, a 'personal choice' we none the less feel that this 'handful' does reflect the richness – be it gravity, élan, or humour – of this country's culture.

Chris Newman   **Nice Nights/Nette Nächte/Les Nuits gentille**

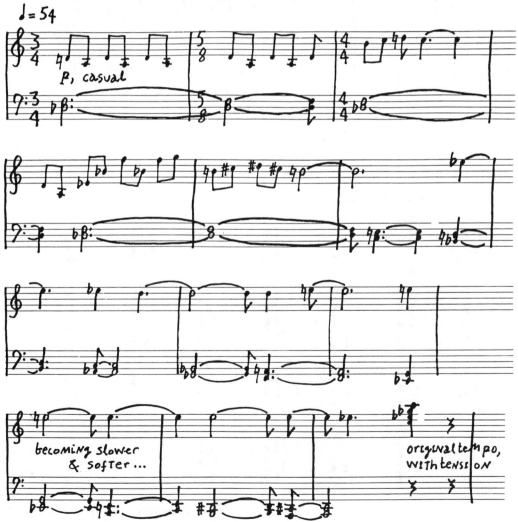

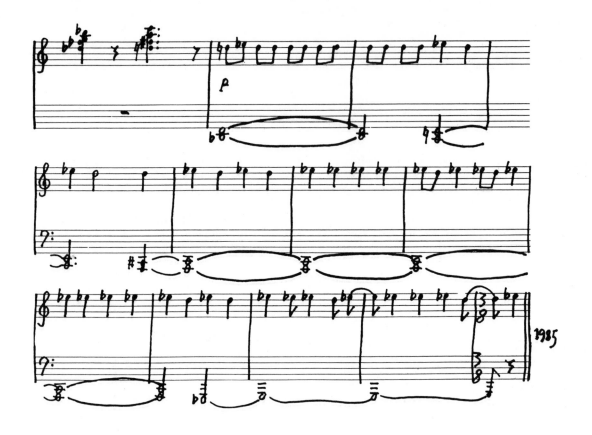

Howard Skempton   **Eirenicon 4 for piano**

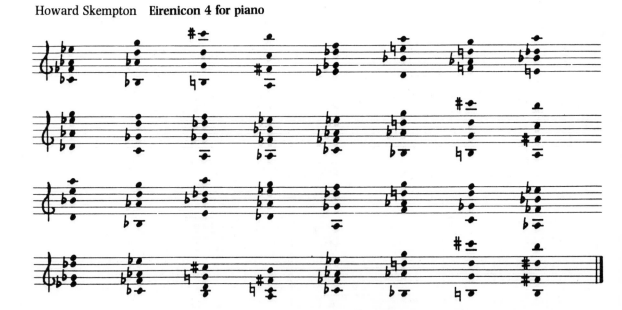

heard

to Martyn Hutchinson and Jonathan Edwards

Richard Barrett

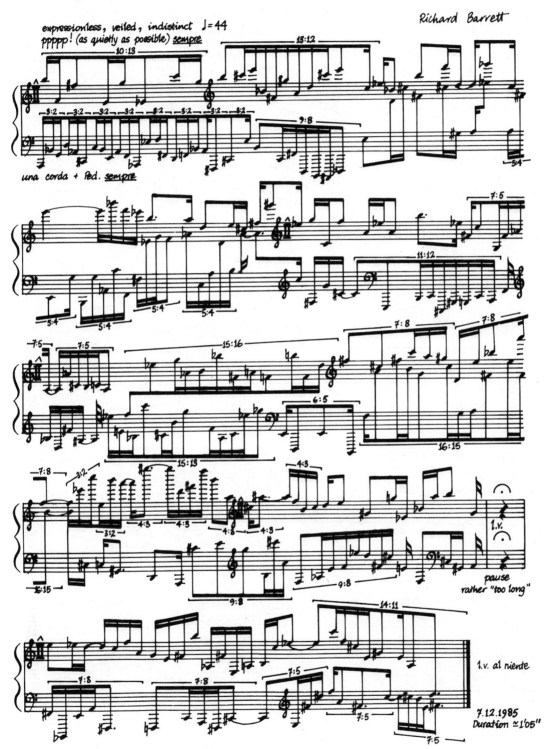

James Dillon **Birl**

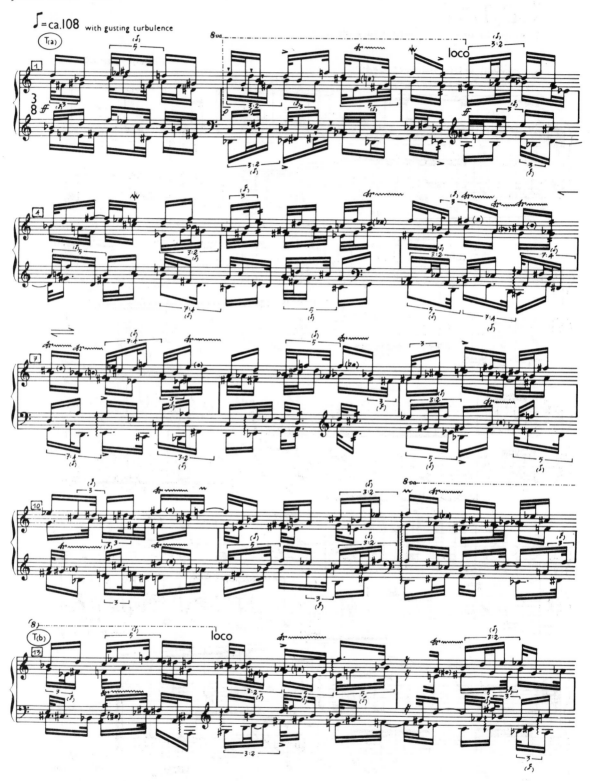

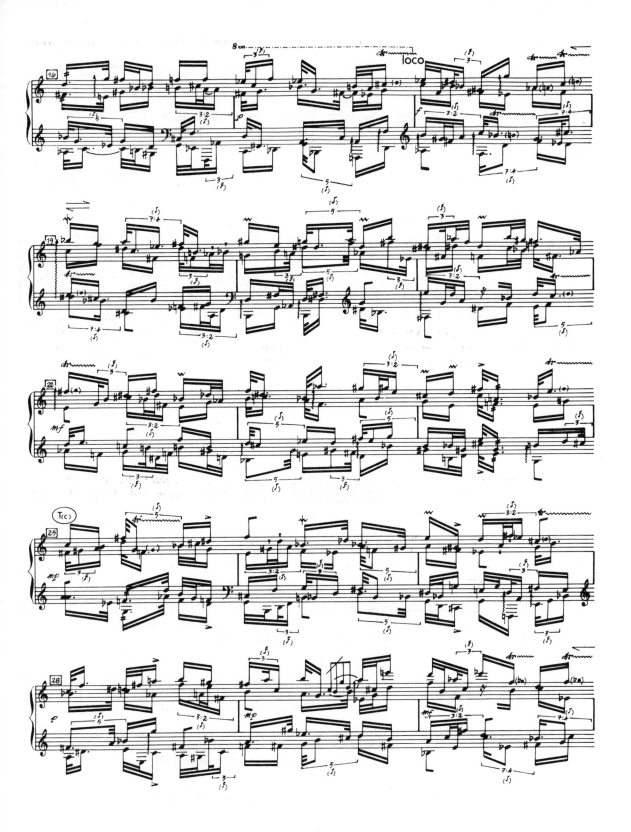

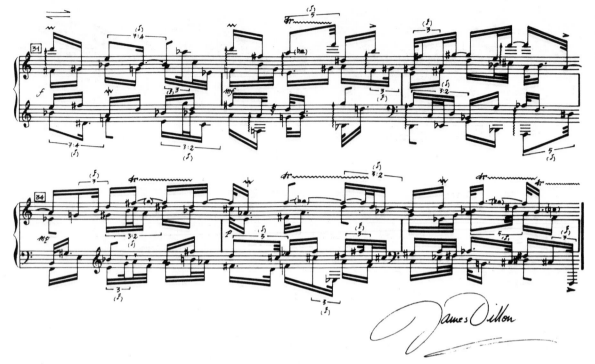

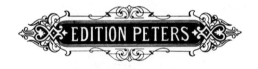

JAMES DILLON

Windows and Canopies (1985)

2Fl, 2Ob, Bsn, 2Hn, Perc, 12Strings
Commissioned by the Gulbenkian Foundation for the Ensemble
Alternance, Paris. Performed in Paris (Oct '85) and Lisbon (May '86)
P-7319. Performing material on hire

Überschreiten (1986)

Fl, Ob, Cl, Bcl, Bsn, Hn, Tpt, Trbn, Tba, Perc, Pf/Org, 2Vln, Vla, Vc, Cb
Commissioned by the Arts Council for the London Sinfonietta
First performed in the Queen Elizabeth Hall, London (June '86)

James Dillon is currently working on an orchestral work, commissioned
by the **BBC** for the **Scottish National Orchestra**, which is to be
performed at **Musica Nova, Glasgow** in **September 1987**

For further information on the works of James Dillon contact
the **Promotion Department, Peters Edition Ltd., 10-12 Baches Street,**
London N1 6DN. Tel: 01-251 6732

Michael's Strathspey

respectfully dedicated to President Finnissy, BMIC

Judith Weir

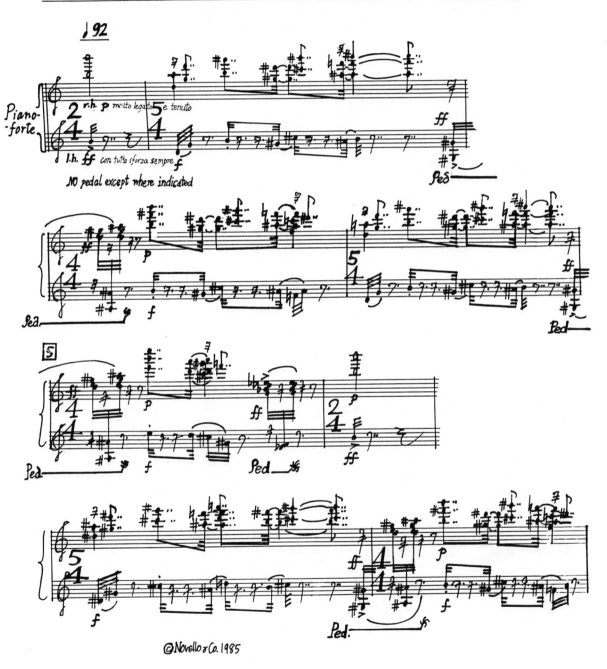

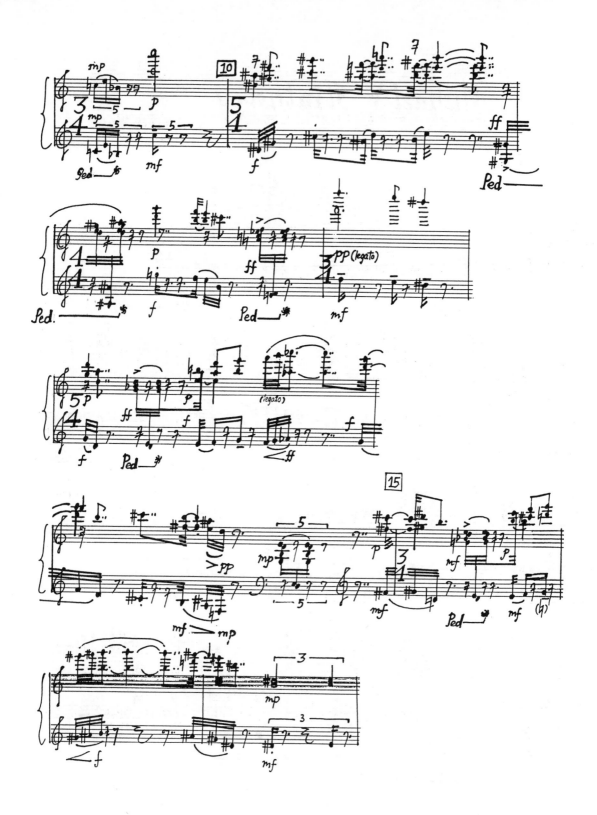

54

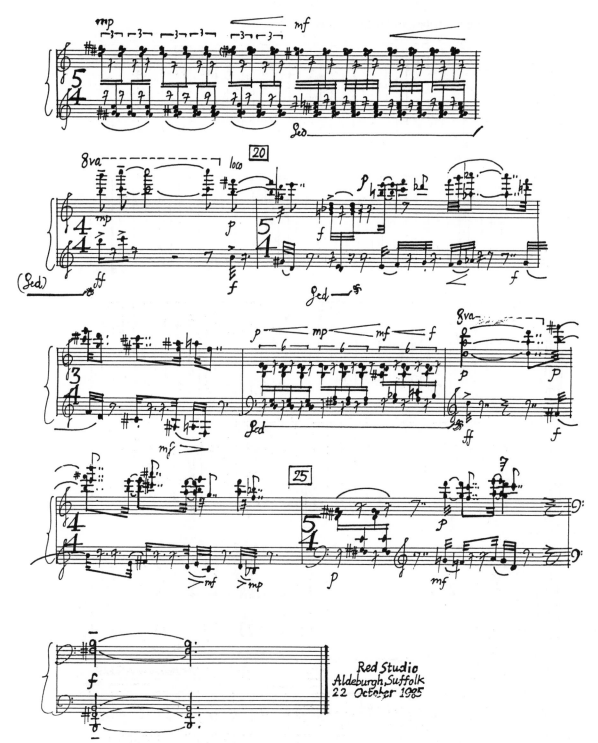

Red Studio
Aldeburgh, Suffolk
22 October 1985

Gerald Barry   Swinging tripes and trillibubkins

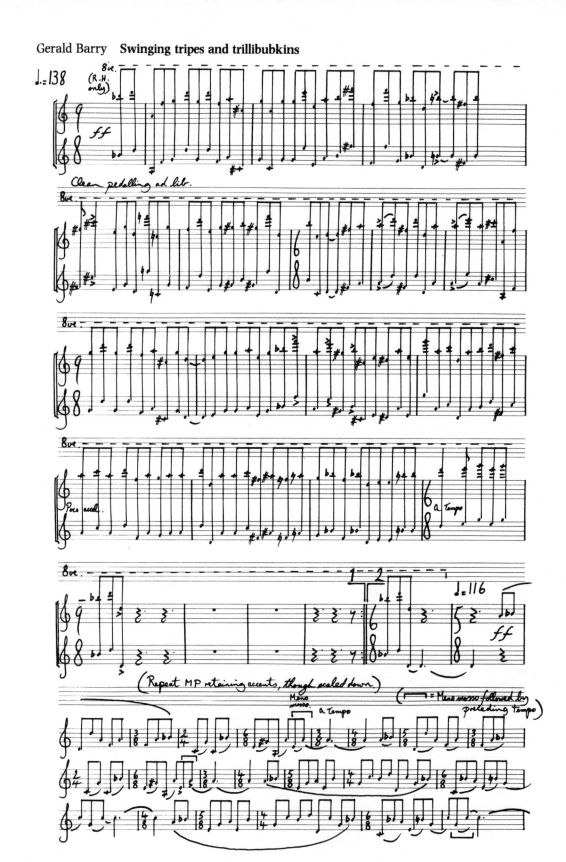

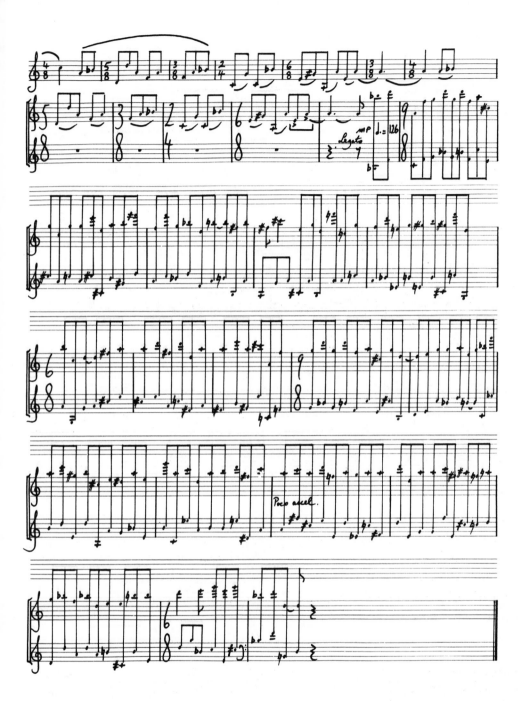

July, 1986.

Michael Finnissy   GFH

Larghetto e piano [♪ = 92 approx.]

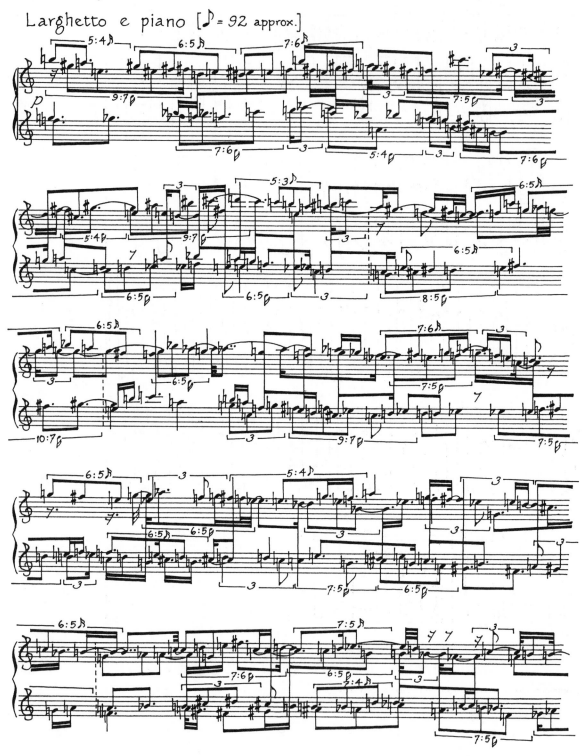

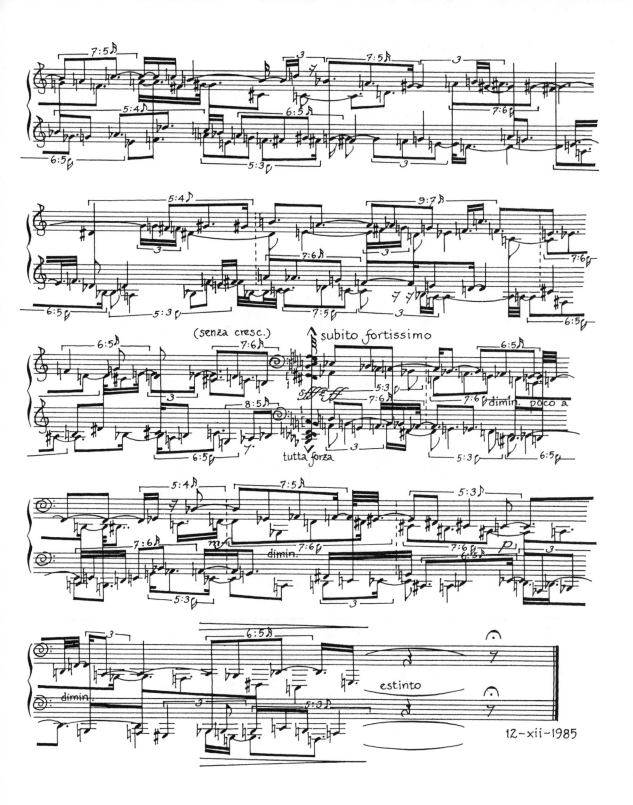

59

Robin Holloway   **Trio from the scherzo giocoso in *Evening with Angels***

Vivace: sotto voce

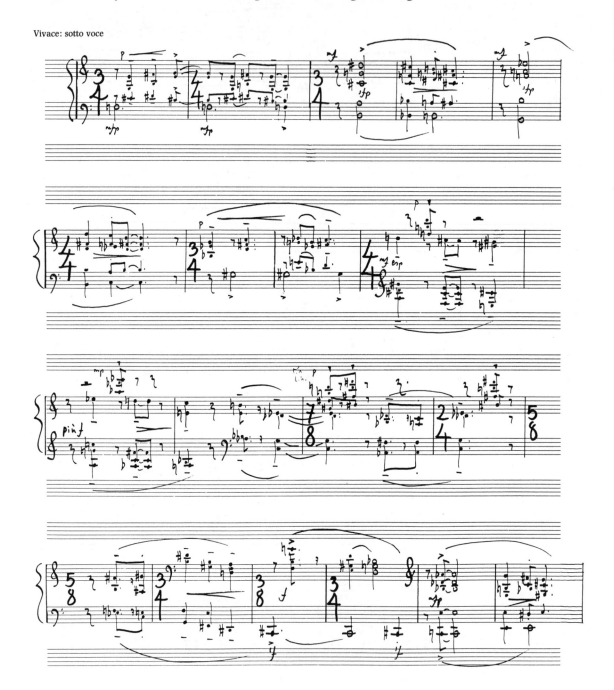

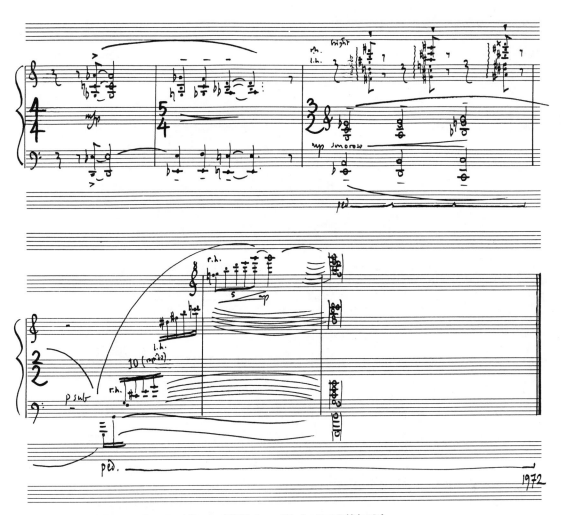

Roger Redgate **Eidos**

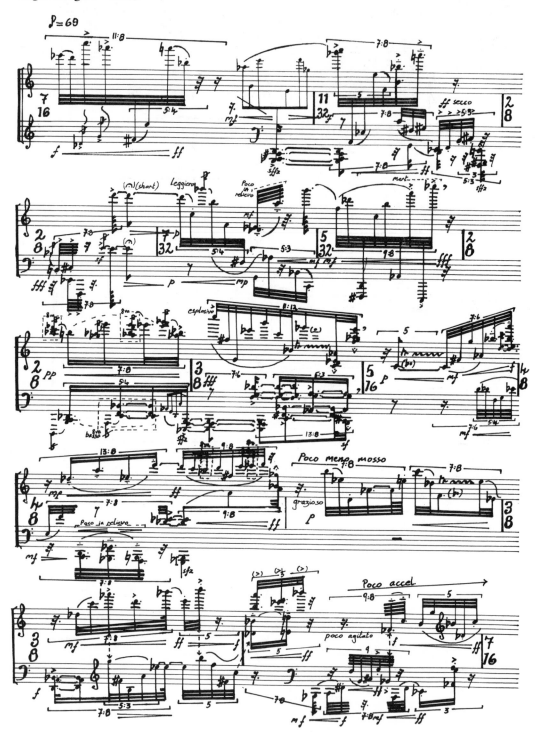

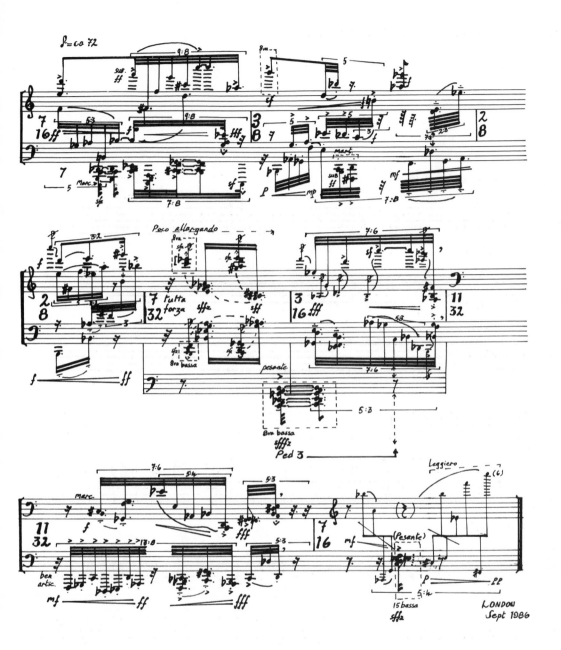

LONDON
Sept 1986

John Tavener   **In Memory of Two Cats (Daisy and Nimrod)**

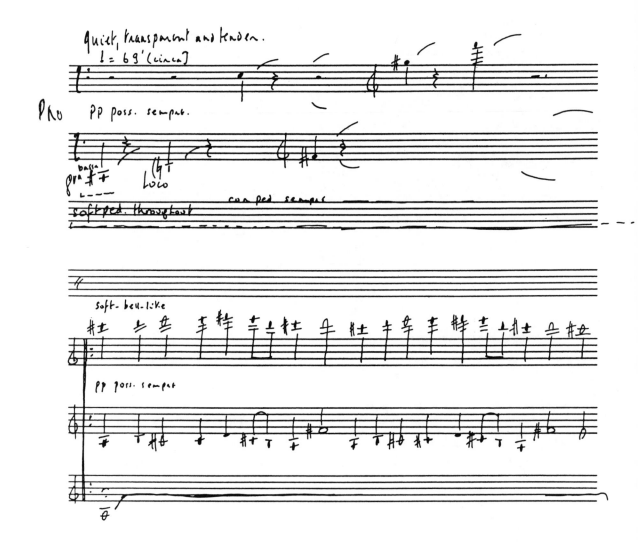

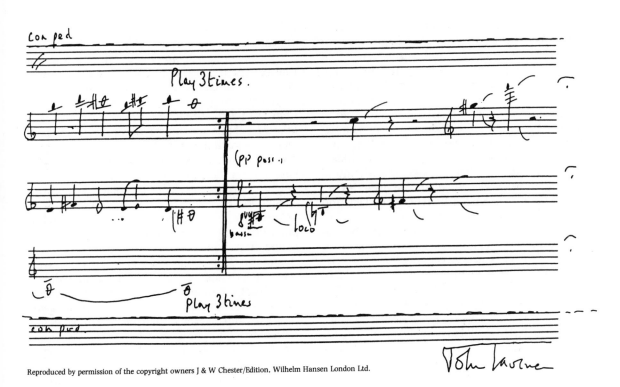

RICHARD TOOP
From Outside Looking in . . .

A view of English music from the other side of the planet has, I suppose, reasonable grounds for claiming to be detached. But if Australia has that detachment, it's relatively recently acquired. After all, the current Master of the Queen's Musick is an Australian, and thanks to the initiatives of publishers like Faber and Universal, it is still easier to buy scores of new Australian music in London than in Sydney and Melbourne. Australian composers of the middle and older generations studied in England with teachers as diverse as Edmund Rubbra, Matyas Seiber, and Peter Maxwell Davies; some of them, like Don Banks, Jennifer Fowler, and David Lumsdaine, chose to stay on.

Conversely, in recent years Australian universities and conservatoires have welcomed English composers like Roger Smalley and Tristram Cary, not to mention a steady trickle of academics (myself included). Until a few years ago, the Australian Broadcasting Corporation was very clearly modelled on a pre-Glock version of the BBC, and although Anglophobia is not quite as comprehensive as it used to be, visits by senior English composers like Alexander Goehr usually manage to set the ABC dovecotes in a flutter, while those by leading expatriates like Lumsdaine pass more or less unnoticed.

Once upon a time, it was more or less self-evident that talented young Australian composers would pursue their studies in England (and not just so as to avoid having to learn a second language). But of late, England has ceased to be the obvious Great Mother: most of our successful young composers (those under 35, let's say) have chosen to study in Europe with, among others, Louis Andriessen, Franco Donatoni, Helmut Lachenmann, and Isang Yun.

So composers' attitudes to English music vary widely according to generation. Nigel Butterley's 50th Birthday Concert included works by his teacher Priaulx Rainier and his spiritual mentor Tippett, while many of the middle generation would still swear by Maxwell Davies (rather than Birtwistle, which I find strange). And in Sydney at least, the younger generation is more inclined to warm to Ferneyhough and Dillon.

In passing, perhaps it's worth pointing out that Australia is one country where the younger generation of composers is not, on the whole, a league of Young Conservatives. As one might infer from their list of teachers, they are pretty well informed about new music in Europe – more so, I would guess, than some young English composers. The New Romanticism is by no means unknown here, but on the whole, it is a cause that has been more readily espoused by the older, established composers (as a sort of second mid-life crisis, to judge from most of the results). So when an English publisher was out here recently, claiming that the young English middle of the road composers were 'filling the Central European gap', his views were received, privately at least, with frank incredulity.

Apart from the differences of emphasis which are self-evident in the notion of personal taste, my own likes and dislikes seem to be very much in line with those of the younger Sydney composers, and I fear they could only distress the bulk of the English musical establishment. In the works of younger composers like Bainbridge, Benjamin, Knussen, Muldowney, and Saxton, I can't hear any substantial trace of the 'breath of fresh air' that the publicists like to talk about: all I can hear is a wilful restoration of the stale old Cheltenham tradition that Birtwistle and Maxwell Davies mercifully began to sweep aside in the late fifties.

The most striking thing about the English 'new romantic' movement has been its total lack of drama: no rampaging Rihms, not even the drastic youth cult of the shell-shocked Schott kiddies (von Bose, Müller-Siemens, *et al.*). Whereas the German version was presented as yet another 'revaluation of all values', the English one looks more like a return to the traditional English values (as opposed to virtues) of understatement and 'good taste'. In fact, the nearest thing to a 'confrontational' New Romanticism in England probably came about twenty years ago, with the première of John Tavener's *In Alium*; and the direction in which

Tavener's music has moved subsequently, away from 'art' towards ritual, has – irrespective of how one regards the musical language – a certain implacable logic. In many ways, there's a striking parallel with the radical simplification one finds in the later work of Henryk Gorecki – the massive *Beatus Vir*, for instance – which is completely detached from 'new music' as such, and yet could probably only have grown out of it. Arvo Pärt's music is another instance of the same phenomenon, and although one could point to the Catholic faith as the decisive factor in all three cases, I can't help feeling that such uncompromising simplicity is really the only honest outcome of any attempt to turn the clock back. The German critic Heinz-Klaus Metzger used to say 'The alternative to complexity is not simplicity, but brutal simplification'. Maybe so: certainly, the current neo-Cheltenham movement seems to me to have no authentic ethos, but simply to stumble from one dismal compromise to the next.

Its reward, of course, is the sanction of officialdom. It seems to be a curiously Anglo-Saxon trait (equally present in Australia!) that one praises one's own conservatives, and other people's radicals. In so far as conservatives, almost by definition, outnumber 'radicals', this is a matter of basic expedience. It's always the same: in order to bolster a country's cultural prestige, the number of 'outstanding composers' is artificially boosted until a situation is reached where, as the Dodo says in *Alice*, '*Everybody* has won, and *all* must have prizes.'

History suggests that the real world of art (if one is permitted the luxury of believing that such a thing exists) isn't like that. In the Vienna of the 1820s there were only two great composers – Beethoven and Schubert, and the whole reputation of the 'classical' era rests on a mere handful of composers. Even through the greatest era of English music – the sixteenth century, with its apparently seamless stream of major figures like Fayrfax, Sheppard, Taverner, Tye, Tallis, Whyte, Byrd, and Gibbons – there were rarely more than two composers at the height of their powers at any one time.

So it is remarkable enough that – as it seems to me – England has two genuinely outstanding composers (Birtwistle and Ferneyhough), a very substantial elder statesman (Tippett), some solid secondary figures (Maxwell Davies, and perhaps Gilbert and Harvey), and a handful of promising youngsters (particularly James Dillon, and others from the group that sprang up around Michael Finnissy). The rest, seen through this particular pair of outside eyes, looks very like nationalist hype.

As in most countries, there have already been significant casualties in the middle generation. What has become of David Bedford, whose work seemed so fresh and promising in the late 60s and early 70s? And the Cardew case remains terribly sad, both personally and musically (Konrad Boehmer's very touching and perceptive memoir of Cardew in the 1984 Donaueschingen brochure is well worth an English translation, if it hasn't already received one). It was Cardew's death, I suppose, that sounded the virtual death-knell of the appealingly eccentric alliance of John Cage with Victorian/Edwardian drawing-rooms that flourished up to the mid-70s under the sobriquet of 'English Experimental Music'. Or does it still exist? Its resolute domesticity and apparent horror of the big gesture (Nyman apart) can't have assisted its passage beyond the English Channel (though the last two discs of Gavin Bryars and Tom Phillips I came across were actually of Franco-Belgian origin). Nor can its intermittent excursions into very woolly (or just plain sheepish?) versions of Marxism have helped, especially when, as with Cardew's last pieces, some excruciatingly banal music made the ideology look more like an alibi than a conviction.

Scarcely less perplexing, to me at any rate, is the increasing conservatism of Maxwell Davies' work, which now seems intent on restoring precisely those Sibelius-plus-Berkeley values that his early pieces rebelled against thirty years ago. I still have vivid memories of hearing one of the first performances of the *Leopardi Fragments* as a teenager at the Dartington Summer School, and it is very hard for me to hear works like the *Sinfonia Concertante* or the *Sinfonietta Accademica* as representing anything remotely like a quarter-century's advance on that marvellous early piece. Being wise after the event, I suppose one could now see the satirical obsessions of many pieces in the 60s as a prediction of conservatism to come (after all, even Bliss and Walton were wild young satirists once), and the cantus firmus technique did have a potentially academic sense of security embedded in it. But there was a time – right up to *A Mirror of Whitening Light* – when the idea of Maxwell Davies as a future Master of the Queen's Musick would have seemed quite bizarre, and now, all of a sudden, it seems terribly plausible.

At the time of the *Leopardi Fragments*, Birtwistle seemed to be a very peripheral figure. How different that looks now! I suppose that what stands out for me in the work of both Birtwistle and

Ferneyhough, despite their discrepancy in style and age, is essentially twofold. One thing is that their music, without undergoing radical stylistic change, is constantly evolving, constantly gaining new dimensions, rather than getting ensnared in expedient routine; despite inevitable local ups-and-downs from one work to the next, their work seems to go on from strength to strength. Ferneyhough's music has interested me ever since I heard a (rather inaccurate) performance of the *Sonata for 2 Pianos* in the late 60s, but for me, the really significant work (perhaps it's a 'middle period') begins as late as 1980, with the second part of *Funérailles*, and *Lemma-Icon-Epigram*, which I have no hesitation in regarding as one of the very few really major piano works since the Boulez sonatas. Birtwistle too seems to have undergone a sort of spiritual regeneration in the late 1970s, at precisely the time when so many others were falling by the wayside. At any rate, pieces like the *Carmen Arcadiae* and *. . . agm . . .* certainly forced me to sharply review *my* attitude to his work, which had previously been one of distant respect rather than actual enthusiasm.

A second factor is that both Birtwistle and Ferneyhough seem to me to be original artists in the true sense of the word: it's not that they imitate no one (which could equally be said of any ignorant amateur), but that they are inimitable. Plenty of young composers have tried (and failed) to imitate them, and will go on trying (and failing).

For this, they receive little official thanks. And in this respect, the output of English record labels tells a fairly significant tale. A label like Lyrita produces a stream of works in the Finzi/Bax/Berkeley mould, but is accessible to living composers, it seems, only upon signing a pact of guaranteed ultra-conservatism. Tippett receives (sometimes rather tardily) the homage due to an elder statesman from the Philips label, and Unicorn does pretty well by Maxwell Davies. Some small independent labels issue occasional discs of works by the 'experimental' faction. The rest, if not quite silence, is a pretty muted whisper. And given the frankly astonishing fact that each of the first three issues in Boulez's *Points de répère* series on the French Erato label includes a work by one of the more adventurous English composers (Birtwistle, Ferneyhough, Harvey), it's hard to see, from outside the chambers of the Arts Council, why British officialdom is quite so hell-bent on neglecting precisely those composers who bring English music some measure of international prestige.

If it's conceded that they *are* English, that is. When I was last in England an Arts Council official asked me in all seriousness whether Ferneyhough, having spent so much time abroad, could really be regarded as an Englishman. As I recollect, John Dowland spent much of his maturity in Denmark, and Peter Philips lived the last thirty years of his life in Brussels. Presumably that same official would prefer to see the works of these unpatriotic renegades expunged from the august volumes of *Musica Britannica*. Even in the closing years of the twentieth century, the British musical establishment seems intent on clinging to a flat earth policy: what you can't see from the cliffs of Dover, doesn't exist.

Seen from the other side of the world, England's official musical culture can look rather like one of Claes Oldenburg's monuments: a huge 'soft monolith', subject to modification only when someone can propose a change that will make it even flabbier. Yet Birtwistle operas do eventually get staged – something inconceivable within the repertoire of the Australian Opera; which was fossilized at birth (we're still waiting for a staging of *Wozzeck*). Maybe one of these days *The Mask of Orpheus* will be performed in Sydney, and Ferneyhough's *Carceri d'Invenzione* cycle in London. And what of the future, what of the 'new blood'? James Dillon, Chris Dench, perhaps Richard Barrett, and some like-minded spirits: *spem in alium nunquam habui.*

JO KONDO AND MICHAEL FINNISSY

View from Japan

Out of the constant flow of foreign musicians visiting this country, Jo Kondo has, of late, become a regular visitor. A recipient of a British Council travelling (research) scholarship this last year, he is one of the leading 'middle generation' composers in Japan, and has received wide acclaim internationally. His performances in London have mostly been at the Almeida Theatre. As revealed in this short interview, he is something of an enthusiast for British music and has organized what he feels to be a few representative performances of it in Japan.

MF   What to Japanese audiences and musicians know about British contemporary composers?

JK   Only a few names. Britten is the most famous. Maxwell Davies and Birtwistle are really only names to a Japanese musician, their *music* is not known very widely. Maybe a few people also know about Cardew. Since Tippett's recent visit he has also been recognized as a sort of 'father figure'. Takemitsu acts as the main 'agent' for the younger composers – so we know a little about Knussen and George Benjamin.

MF   Are the current stylistic trends, in as much as they can be recognized or so generalized, similar here to Japan?

JK   Some tendencies are certainly similar. The 'New Romanticism' is quite popular, although the Japanese have had more exposure to the German version of this 'style' – von Bose, Müller Siemens, for example – so they are closer to this than perhaps the British are. There is almost no 'minimalism' – I find that the American experimental tradition couldn't find any roots in Japan, and although some American composers, especially Reich and Riley, are popular with listeners, almost no composers follow their example. There is no music of the type called 'New Complexity'.

MF   Can you compare the quality and quantity of music – new music especially – performed here in London, with Tokyo?

JK   The general quality in London is very, very high – compared even with a city like New York, never mind Tokyo. I don't think Tokyo or New

York have such high standards. Even in the busiest part of the season in Tokyo we still only have three or four concerts per week, in London you have that every day!

MF   How do concerts here differ in preparation or the effect they have on audiences?

JK   Things are not very different in this respect. Possibly you get *more* support from your Government than we do in Japan. The audiences here seem more mixed in age range – in Japan the audience for new music consists entirely of young people. Over a 10-year period this is very depressing, because the public never sticks with you, and never grows ... just a constantly changing audience of the young, who – incidentally – also treat new music very much as a 'fashion', something which is essentially impermanent.

MF   Are many of the younger Japanese composers (40 and under) commercially recorded?

JK   By such means as self-promotion, we have a system like CRI in the States, probably five or so – composers paying for their own records. Some organizations occasionally produce a record as part of a commission 'deal', though these tend to be poor quality live recordings of public concerts, not studio recordings.

MF   And publishing?

JK   Very bad in Japan. Zen On do the older composers (over 50) and University academics. Japanese Schott have taken Takemitsu, Takahashi, and Ichiyanagi. This area is poorer even than recordings. The usual story is that there is *no market*.

MF   You have your own ensemble – Musica Practica – how much British music do you perform?

JK   Generally not much. We did a Birtwistle piece, and then more recently a whole festival: Music Now in London. The festival was supported by the city of Yokohama, where the provincial government are very keen to promote modern Art – Yokohama is the next largest city to Tokyo and they are very competitive. We also got support for the festival from the British Council, enabling us to fly out Gavin Bryars and Simon Holt, and pay for the music hire. In addition to Holt and Bryars we played Finnissy, Saxton, Osborne, and John White. The events were very well received, audiences of 800 people making an enthusiastic response. The concerts were free. NHK Radio recorded three 50-minute programmes.

MF How easy is it to hear or purchase British music in Japan?

JK Most of the broadcasting of new music is based upon an exchange of tapes between NHK and the EBU. Because the BBC do not supply tapes under this scheme we hear almost no British music at all, unless it is via tapes supplied by other countries from festivals. I think this is unfortunate, and it obviously limits a main source of information. Scores are available for sale, since most of the publishers in London have agents in Japan: but I don't think scores sell very well, simply because the names of the composers are not known.

MF Tell me more about 'Musica Practica'.

JK I do all the organizing myself. The musicians – twenty in all – play without fee. It took me 3 years to contact and persuade musicians to do this . . . they otherwise play as studio or session musicians, University teachers, orchestral players, one clarinettist who is a gardener – but they have no other opportunity to play *new* serious music, and they welcomed the chance I was offering. Hire of the venue, and instrument or percussion hire is paid for by ticket sales – we operate on a very narrow margin there! The publisher of my books, I have no publisher in Japan for my music, pays for the programme and brochure printing. The instrumental line-up is similar to the London Sinfonietta, and we are the only large-scale group like that in Japan. Also most of the smaller new music ensembles still insist on a constant flow of 'premières', whereas we do repeats. I believe in programming new work with Varèse, Schoenberg, even Boulez – these composers have a 'classic' status – and I include one 'classic' in each concert (Ives is another composer I have often included); the rest comes from the 1950s or more recent years. We do three or four concerts a year, and it is my intention not to perform and benefit Jo Kondo but to enrich the Japanese Music Scene, thus few concerts feature my work.

MF Do you know of any British composers, or music of interest, that should be more widely advertised?

JK I think *all* British composers should be better known than they seem to be. Even though the general level of skill, quality, and musical concepts is very, very high I find it difficult to focus on any one particular feature as a predominant characteristic. Even though British composers place less emphasis on the purely novel or shocking, their music is very rich in ideas.

MF Do you find our 'ideas' or philosophy all that different?

JK No. There are some strong connections and similarities to the general aesthetic viewpoint in Japan. Both cultures express an interest in extramusical elements, so that even in 'abstract' composition there is still a tendency towards literary derivation. Your art too seems preoccupied with descriptions of Nature, and particularly with a sort of poeticism (literature again!), even though there are obvious differences in the quality and type of image being referred to.

MALCOLM HAYES

Douglas Young's *Ludwig* and some London Dance Events

It still gets put around in some quarters (particularly in operatic ones) that ballet can't be a vehicle for serious ideas. In fact the post-60s British scene seems to regard serious ideas of any kind, even with a small 's', as something fairly close to heresy. Fortunately there are some gifted individuals in the world of dance who are sufficiently independent minded to be able to treat such attitudes with the contempt they deserve. But I don't think it's altogether a coincidence that the most ambitious ballet I've seen in the past year – possibly the strongest, certainly the boldest – was mounted not in Britain but in Germany.

Ludwig, with music by Douglas Young and choreography by Ronald Hynd, was premièred at the Bavarian State Opera in Munich on 14 June 1986 to mark the centenary of the death of King Ludwig II. Its large two-act design, subtitled 'Fragments of a Mystery', charts the confused and ultimately tragic life of the young king; it also represents the first time that a British composer has been commissioned to write for the main theatre of this celebrated and beautiful opera house, which gave the first performances of Wagner's *Tristan*, *Meistersinger*, *Rheingold*, and *Walküre* as well as of several of Richard Strauss's operas. Many of the events depicted in the ballet actually happened within the building, while others, such as the liaison between Wagner and Cosima von Bülow, certainly occurred nearby.

Ludwig II succeeded to the Bavarian throne in 1864 when he was only 18, and from the start his imagination and sensitivity found themselves hopelessly at odds with the trappings of the life he had to lead. *Ludwig* is the reverse, then, of ballet masquerading as pageant: here music, choreography, and design all set out to explore the deepening incompatibility between the private individual and his official role, tracing the sequence of Ludwig's unstable relationships with Wagner, Prince Paul, and Princess Sophie against the background of the loneliness of his inner mind, and moving relentlessly towards the mysterious circumstances of his

death by drowning in the Starnbergersee. The ballet succeeds outstandingly because it is conceived as a totality and comes across as such – Wagner's concept of the *Gesamtkunstwerk*, if you like, working itself out in a different medium. Of course there are individual moments which don't yet work, but they are easily swept aside by the spectacular achievement of the whole. I have not seen such a bold mixture of elements pull together in exactly this way since the Cologne Opera production of Zimmermann's *Die Soldaten* at the 1972 Edinburgh Festival.

Douglas Young's score, though instrumental in origin, is entirely on tape: the music was realized by Young and Tryggvi Tryggvason at the electronic studios of East Anglia University, a 16-track master then being made at the Staatsoper. The prospect of an empty orchestra pit and an array of loudspeakers for the whole of a full-length ballet might have seemed unappetizing, but in fact the music compels both on its own terms and in the context of the staging. With no disrespect to Hynd's choreography, the work's structure is essentially generated by the music and in particular by Young's skilful transitions between the scenes – a Wagnerian technique if ever there was one. Much of the material is derived from themes from Wagner's operas (later also from Liszt's *Lugubre gondola* pieces); Young develops these in a manner which brings them into his own sound-world, a high-risk strategy which on the whole succeeds remarkably, the end result being anything but derivative. To be able to sustain a score of this size with these methods indicates a sharply focused imagination and a degree of technical strength which I suspect few composers could approach.

The tone is set by Ludwig's appearance in Act I, Scene i, accompanied by a single probing cello line which is, in fact, the first phrase that Lohengrin sings in his eponymous opera – 'Nun sei gedankt, mein lieber Schwan' – transposed an octave lower: it sounds at once the same and quite

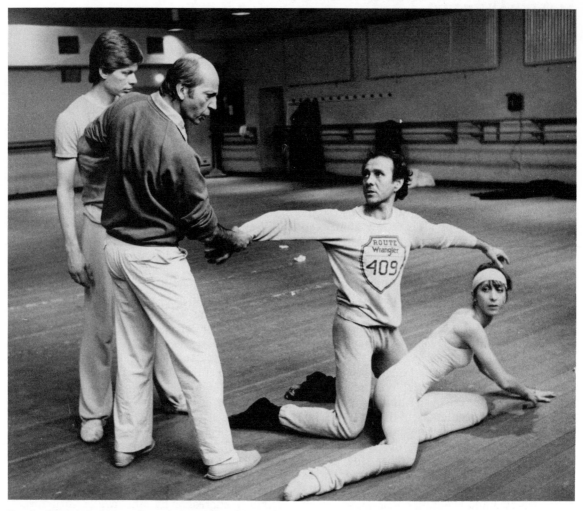

Douglas Young's *Ludwig* in rehearsal – Ronald Hynd (second from left), with Ferenc Barbay (Wagner) and Jolinda Menendez (Cosima)

different. The cello is the perfect instrument to characterize Ludwig, and it also gives Young the opportunity to make maximum use of some superlative playing by Rohan de Saram. Other fine passages include a five-part fantasia on Hans Sachs's theme from Act III of *Meistersinger* for the duet between Wagner and Ludwig, and a development (harmonically speaking) of 'Träume', the fifth of the *Wesendonck Lieder*, for Wagner and Cosima. Pastiche is a world away except where specifically intended: the opening scene of Act II is a Ball at the Residenz, Ludwig's palace in Munich, and the quadrille with which it begins finds Young cheerfully parodying Chabrier's own take-off of Wagner in his *Souvenirs de Munich*. Throughout, electronic techniques as such – sound-transformation, montage, spatial deployment – are used

with a judicious restraint which makes them all the more effective.

Taking a cue from Young's music, Hynd's choreography is similarly rich in allusions which enhance rather than mask its own inventiveness. This came across clearly in the sequence of duets in Act I: I have not seen enough of Béjart's work to be sure that the passages for Ludwig and Wagner, and later Ludwig and Prince Paul, related to it as much as they seemed to, but the Wagner-Cosima duet directly invoked the MacMillan style, if anything outdoing it for charged eroticism, while the tentative relationship between Ludwig and Sophie recalled Ashton at his most delicate. (Incidentally Ferenc Barbay, Jolinda Menendez, and Deborah Weiss as – respectively – Wagner, Cosima, and Sophie, each looked so like their original counterparts that I began to speculate as to what kind of occult forces might be at work.) Both composer and choreographer are agreed that Act I needs to be tightened up a little, but to my mind the contrasts in Act II of big set-pieces with the scenes of Ludwig's increasing isolation were just about faultlessly paced. Munich Ballet may not have a reputation as a front-line company but I think anyone would have been impressed by the strength and conviction of the dancing in the performance I saw (the last of the scheduled six): Jan Broeckx was outstanding in the huge role of Ludwig, and I especially liked Deborah Weiss's demure yet anxious portrayal of Sophie.

Bernd-Dieter Müller's designs and Rudolf Rappmansberger's lighting featured the occasional oddity but also found room for some brilliant ideas: the use of back-lit slide-projection was far more adventurous than we tend to see over here. Indeed the whole production was redolent of a sensible amount of money sensibly spent. Bavarian audiences may not be tuned in to ballet as British ones are, but the familiarity of the subject will have helped, and word had obviously got around that here was something to come and see; the applause

at the end was sustained and sincere. The Staatsoper has scheduled *Ludwig* for revival in the summer of 1987, although plenty can happen to ballet schedules over a 12-month period!

Choreographic activity on this side of the Channel continued as busily as ever during the year. Rather than reel off a shopping-list of titles, I'll mention two in particular where the musical component was unusually interesting.

David Bintley's *The Sons of Horus* was originally commissioned by Paris Opéra Ballet and was about half-way complete in rehearsal there in early 1985 before the production was cancelled, officially due to 'lack of rehearsal time' ('political sabotage' would seem to be closer to the mark). Fortunately the Royal Ballet scheduled six performances in October and November 1985; Bintley must have thought his ballet was permanently jinxed when some of *those* were cancelled due to the orchestral strike, although a second run of performances did in fact follow later in the season. I saw the work in November and again in April and on both occasions came away much impressed with Peter McGowan's specially written score.

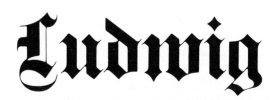

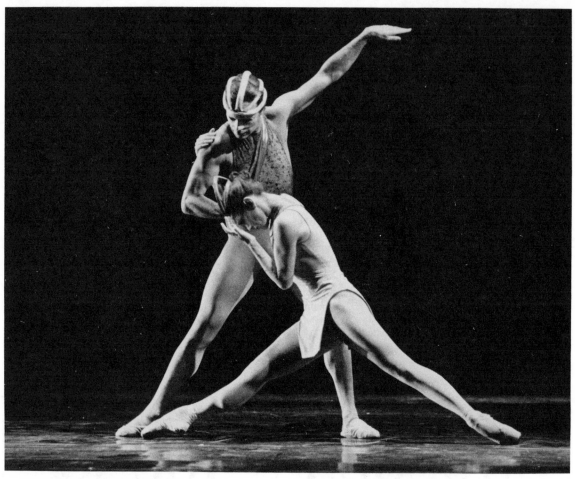

Scene from David Bintley's *The Sons of Horus*

Bintley and McGowan had together worked out a scenario which was both evocative in mood and precisely structured – the ideal blend for this kind of one-act design. In ancient Egyptian mythology, the four Sons of Horus were minor deities whose principal task was the protection of certain parts of the body after death, one of the processes that was believed to be essential if the dead person's soul was to enter the afterlife in the 'Field of Reeds', and said to have been invented by Isis for her dead husband Osiris. The ballet's outline, then, is basically a sequence of four contrasted set-pieces centred round each of the four Sons of Horus in turn – the falcon-headed Qebhsnuf, the ape-headed Hapi, the human-headed Imsety, and the jackal-headed Duamutef – placed within and linked by a ritual framework whose material is first introduced in the Prelude ('Isis mourns'). Each of these four main movements uses a different musical form, respectively sonata form, scherzo and trio, an arpeggiated variant of the opening

Ritual, and a set of variations; the latter are punctuated by 'mini-rituals' of their own, out of the last of which flows the final section, the 'Journey to the Field of Reeds'.

The world of ancient myth is thus imaged in a carefully balanced structure, and the allusion to Stravinsky could hardly be more direct nor, in this case, more gracefully articulated by composer and choreographer alike. McGowan builds his score out of the simplest of elements with absolute expertise – the curling unaccompanied eight-note arabesque for solo oboe at the very start, for instance, is then verticalized into a pair of four-note chords, these two complementary ideas instantly defining the music's sound-world. The underlying mood is both sombre and serene (the omission of violins and violas from the scoring at once recalls the *Symphony of Psalms*), but the subtle rhythmic presence makes for a nicely danceable idiom; the different characters of the four set-pieces are sharply projected, and then the final 'Journey' unfolds on a stream of overlapping repetitive phrase-patterns. McGowan mentions that he has 'the experience of our contemporary "minimalist" music in mind', but I think he does himself an injustice if he is referring to the rhythmic and harmonic banality of Reich or Glass: his own idiom here, on the contrary, is beautifully poised in both respects. The 'Journey to the Field of Reeds' is really no more 'minimalist' than the opening of the fourth tableau of *Petrushka*.

Bintley's choreography blends the hieratic gestures of Egyptian wall-painting into the syntax of classical ballet to memorable effect – I'm thinking in particular of the opening Prelude for Isis, marvellously executed by Lesley Collier. The final 'Journey' hauntingly mirrors McGowan's music in a tranced unbroken processional for the entire cast from left to right of the stage, with Ashley Page's Duamutef (if I remember rightly) contributing the occasional anarchic little cross-current. Terry Bartlett's designs are both austere and atmospheric, as is John B. Read's lighting. Two thoughts: first (fervently) that *The Sons of Horus* remains in the Royal Ballet's repertory for a long time to come, and second, that McGowan's score finds its way onto record (it deserves it).

Christopher Bannerman's *Shadows In The Sun* was premièred by London Contemporary Dance Theatre in Nottingham in September 1985, meeting with a mixed critical reception; I saw it in LCDT's December season at Sadler's Wells and couldn't understand such a faint-hearted response (I still don't). The work is loosely based on D. H. Lawrence's novel *Women In Love*, evoking the Lawrentian world of fluctuating human relationships in universal rather than overly specific terms. I fail to see why this puzzled people – what's wrong with a 'mood' ballet? After all, no one criticizes *Les Sylphides* for being 'vague' (do they?). Granted that Andrew Storer's design – a single door leading to nowhere in particular, set in a nondescript pink background – had an air of obscurity; granted too that there were uneven moments in Bannerman's choreography, but the best of it was most beautiful. It was also, of course, quite superbly danced: memory lingers on a duet for Brenda Edwards – wonderfully quick and lithe – and Kenneth Tharp.

But what really struck me was Bannerman's instinct for choosing the right music. The composer one would first think of as being closest to Lawrence would be Delius – the glowing, epic trajectory of *The Rainbow*, for instance, relates immediately to the warm colours and the great spaces of the *Mass of Life*. But *Women In Love* is a quite different conception – conversational, elliptically constructed, with an intellectual, even dialectical streak. Frank Bridge's later music mirrors this side of Lawrence perfectly in its probing mercurial unease, its beauty of syntax articulating a world of almost desperate instability. Bannerman's selection – *Elegy, Morning Song, Solitude, Water Nymphs,* and parts of the Second Piano Trio – made a lovely little chamber ballet of its own; the silences interspersed between the pieces, during which the characters literally and psychologically regrouped themselves, were here a telling contribution in their own right rather than the contemporary-dance cliché they can sometimes become. Bridge's music also demands skilled execution which was duly provided by Nicola Lewis (violin), Caroline Dale (cello), and LCDT's company pianist Eleanor Alberga, the latter rippling through Bridge's iridescent keyboard figuration with suppleness and fluency.

Finally, Susan Crow's *Track and Field* demands more than just an honourable mention. Premièred in Eastbourne on 13 December 1985 by Sadler's Wells Royal Ballet (I saw it in London a few weeks later), it took Degas's famous painting *Young Spartans* as a starting-point for a witty and ingenuous little *Agon* for four girls and four men – honours even at the end, naturally! Crow's inventive and appealing choreography was enhanced by her interesting choice of music, the American composer David Diamond's *Rounds* for string orchestra – neo-classical in style but none the less strongly characterized, and of course brim-full of crisp danceable rhythms. Graham Lustig's *Caught in Time*, danced to Walter Leigh's astringent little *Concertino* for harpsichord and strings and created under the same tight conditions as Crow's work, was almost as good. It's remarkable what can be achieved on a budget of just £1,000 if the necessary talent is there.

TOM MORGAN

Birtwistle's *The Mask of Orpheus*

1986 was undoubtedly an extraordinary year in the career of Harrison Birtwistle. The London Sinfonietta took *Secret Theatre* (1984), one of its finest commissions, on a nationwide tour. The BBC Symphony Orchestra gave the première in March of the large-scale and enormously impressive *Earth Dances*. David Freeman and Elgar Howarth were both involved in the first performances of two major stage works. In August, Opera Factory produced *Yan Tan Tethera* (1984), and in May English National Opera unveiled a work we had been awaiting more than a decade, *The Mask of Orpheus*. Over five hours of music by a composer in impressive form was heard for the first time!

The importance of this has not gone unrecognized. There have been mini Birtwistle festivals in York and London, the Baylis Programme ran an educational project around *The Mask of Orpheus*, while radio talks, articles anticipating the new works, unusually long reviews, and even colour supplement profiles of the composer, all testified to an abnormally high level of public interest. Even the 'hedgehog-like' composer himself uncurled to advise on the production of his offspring and give public talks and interviews, and gave us an occasional glimpse of his serious and lucid thoughts usually hidden beneath his gruff exterior. Is it possible, that, with a sense of the importance of these works, he has gained some of the confidence that distinguishes two of his more outgoing and articulate colleagues in the former New Manchester School?

Of the three new works, *The Mask of Orpheus* understandably received most attention. Its long gestation, its almost legendary libretto, rumours of productions at Covent Garden and Glyndebourne, interest in Barry Anderson's electronic music, the chapter in Michael Hall's book,[1] all fuelled interest. Frequent reference to Birtwistle's work as an 'opera' and its production in a conventional opera house may have reinforced misconceptions about the nature of the work. Birtwistle's own description of 'Lyric Tragedy', though apt in a sense, arouses confusing associations with the French Eighteenth Century. The work needs a more helpful subtitle to relate it to the ritualistic traditions of Greek classical drama and perhaps to the stylized world of the English masque.

.   When expectations run high, misconceptions are likely to occur and it is almost inevitable that some should express disappointment and reservations. Even so, *The Mask of Orpheus* received a careful and thoughtful press, unlike Nigel Osborne's opera *Hell's Angels*, first performed in January 1986, which provoked the critics to indulge in a shameful orgy of ill-considered comment and personal abuse.

Perhaps the most serious criticism of Birtwistle's work was that it is essentially undramatic. Many preferred the more traditional narrative and goal-directed dramatic structure of the central act, in which Orpheus dreams of his journey in Hades through seventeen arches to retrieve Euridice. (No wonder that this sensational music will form the basis of a concert suite.) Impressive as this act is, to suggest that the work as a whole, and the outer acts in particular, is undramatic is to miss or reject the work's special dramatic character. Even before the subject was chosen, Birtwistle, with characteristic lucidity, recognized that the nature of his musical language would lead him to an unusual concept of drama. 'At the time I was working with forms of repetition, blocks that are repeated from different angles but are never the same.' This is one of the central concerns of much of his music. For a suitable theatrical counterpart he chose, after rejecting Faust, the legend of Orpheus, and turned to Peter Zinovieff for a libretto.

This ancient legend has fascinated composers since the time of Monteverdi, and Birtwistle is no exception, witness its appearance in works such as *Nenia* (1970) and the recent choral work *On the Sheer Threshold of the Night* (1980). One reason it suited Birtwistle was that there are several versions. By utilizing, sometimes consecutively, sometimes even concurrently, the different points of view of the story, the libretto corresponds to that

1   Michael Hall, *Harrison Birtwistle* (London, Robson Books Ltd, 1984), pp. 114–42.

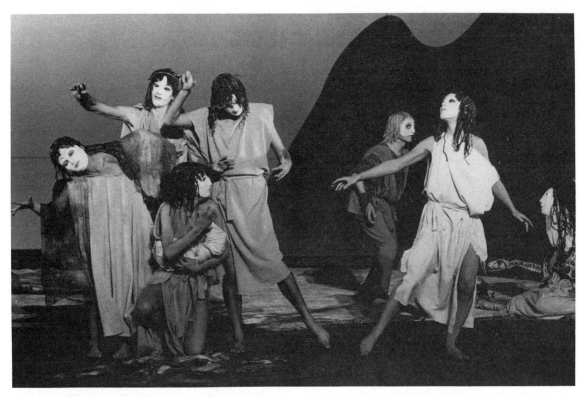

Scene from Harrison Birtwistle's *The Mask of Orpheus*

essential element of repetition in Birtwistle's musical language. The risk of confusion of such a complex apparatus is alleviated by the audience's familiarity with at least one version of the story. There is no suspense of 'finding out' what happens. It is a drama not of discovery or development, but of experience and re-experience and re-examination from different perspectives. Some have applied the term 'cubist'; nor is it far removed from the notion of ritual.

This cubist concept is reinforced by the daring device of representing Orpheus, Euridice, and Aristaeus each by three people. A singer represents the man or woman, a puppet (who also sings) represents the character as 'Myth', and a mime represents the 'hero'. The same events may thus be seen from the human, mythic, or heroic points of view.

Zinovieff's unusual libretto is a fascinating, though at times obscure artefact. It contains much that is confusing or difficult to accept. The naïvety or obscurity of sections of the text, the use of an invented language, the density of events, their elaborate labelling and complex groupings, the devices of time shift, the different structures for each act (particularly the 'Tide' structure of the third), and the mass of charts, tables, and explanatory notes all seem perverse and pretentious. And superficially at least, it seems by conventional standards unpromising material for the stage, even essentially undramatic.

However, if one bears in mind the composer's comments about the nature of his music and note that his collaboration with Zinovieff set out to parallel these qualities in the libretto, many of these objections and reservations lose their force. The libretto quite deliberately provides a highly stylized, ritualized framework of repeated events, words, and images. Birtwistle complements them in his remarkable music.

Even so, such a suggestive libretto has stimulated a wonderfully *fluid* response from the composer. Each of the libretto's many gestures and events is articulated by a change in the music, so that (cross-related) discrete blocks gradually accumulate into an enormous structure. Both libretto and music are obsessed with repetition, though in different ways. The wonder is that the music has, despite its block structure, a remarkable continuity and momentum. It is a rare example of a long, slowly paced work justifying itself by the quality of invention and consistency of execution. A powerful technical means, which Birtwistle has developed over the years, ensures this sense of continuity.

Birtwistle has long regarded 'monody' as an essential dimension of his music. But in recent years, particularly in *Secret Theatre* and *The Mask of Orpheus*, it has become more striking and supple, especially when enriched by a kind of 'organum' technique. The harmony too seems richer. It seems not just concerned with filling in the chromatic space between two notes, but has developed a more distinctive character through a more careful choice of notes. Rhythmically, Birtwistle's music has always been very interesting. The music of Act III shows that in the years since the completion of Act II, his language has developed an arresting, punchy aspect, which we have also heard in works like *Carmen Arcadiae . . .* and *Earth Dances*, and which in *The Mask of Orpheus* becomes a powerful means of generating momentum and tension. If at times the most disappointing and least interesting aspect of the music is the vocal writing, it does at least throw one's attention onto the large wind and percussion orchestra and onto the most striking achievement of the work, namely the electronic music.

The highly experienced Barry Anderson provided the technical expertise (which Birtwistle himself lacked) for this part of the score. More significantly, as a composer in his own right, he was able to take much of the responsibility for the actual composition of the extensive electronic music, though regrettably this is frequently acknowledged only as an afterthought. To some extent, the electronic music replaced the blending and background function of the missing string section, and the background 'auras' added to the sense of continuity. The strength of his contribution, however, was most apparent during the mimed 'panels' which interrupted the main action, where we were treated to a feast of purely electronic sound.

Another important feature of his work was the subtle and flexible inter-relationship of the live and electronic musics. At times, voices and instruments were heard alone, but because all the voices and sections of the orchestra were amplified through loudspeakers, the barrier between 'human' and 'mechanical' music was broken. The fusion went further, and not only because of the closeness of the collaboration between the two composers. The actual choice of material for electronic modification was largely based on the harp and human voice. This meant that the electronic music was related to the 'live' sounds at a fundamental level. Anderson's real achievement was to produce music which was self-effacing or richly imaginative and compelling as the context demanded. He 'lost' his own personality or impressed us with the strength of his creativity only when appropriate.

Zinovieff, Birtwistle, and Anderson have created a striking and unusual kind of theatre, that for all its problems has a fundamental integrity of conception and execution. It prefers reflection to narration and ritual to realism. Unfortunately David Freeman's production, for all his ability to produce very striking, simple, memorable images, failed to complement these essential qualities. Like so many modern productions, he did not allow the action to grow out of the music. His ideas appeared to come from a free re-interpretation of the libretto alone, though even then he ignored vital suggestions. The result was at times a profusion of unnecessary and distracting detail; at others, a poverty of visual information. It was fortunate that the music was so strong. At times Freeman responded with stylized action of the wrong kind, and frequently the production was too realistic and contradicted the essentially ritualistic nature of the work.

Ultimately, however, the richness of the work overcame the poverty of the production, for at successive performances it revealed new dimensions, to a degree that the present writer has not experienced before. This confirms the fascination of the work and reinforces its 'cubist' preoccupation with re-experiencing the same events from different perspectives. The power and excitement it generated demonstrated palpably that such a static, ritualistic, and cubist conception can make good theatre. However unorthodox, it convinces us that it is essentially dramatic.

There are indications that a revival is being contemplated at the London Coliseum, but not for another four years. When it comes it is to be hoped that the formidable talents of Philip Langridge, Barry Anderson, and conductors Elgar Howarth and Paul Daniel amongst others are reassembled, as the musical side of the production was of a consistently high standard. Meanwhile other houses should be urged to programme it soon, for further productions are needed to reveal yet more dimensions of this rich and complex work.

BARRIE GAVIN

New Music and TV – Bridging the Gap

'Bridge that gap with a Cadbury's snack' – thus quipped a TV advert from the 1970s. Today, if there is something of a chasm between audiences and the new music of our time, then it is my belief that television has a role to play in building a bridge across that chasm.

It is a coincidence (but a happy one) that I am writing this in a hotel in the little German town of Donaueschingen. Most of the year it produces beer, but for a few days every October it produces, in the 'Donaueschinger Musiktage', the newest of new music. So these thoughts on the televising of contemporary music come between bouts of wrestling with a camera script which will somehow cope with the torrential complexity of Brian Ferneyhough's 'Carceri d'Invenzione'. It is, at least in the beginning, a logistic problem. How can one best reflect the character and structure of a piece from a strictly limited number of visual viewpoints? Well, a string quartet and four cameras might initially seem a well-balanced form of combat, but even then the music will throw up a far richer series of relationships, both precise and ambiguous, than can be adequately represented by the television director. Instead he has to seek a kind of parallel structure, which will somehow provide the watching audience with a pictorial metaphor for the aural experience. New music, perhaps fortunately, does not lend itself readily to record-sleeve symbolism – passing clouds, misty mountains, the inevitable sunlight through trees. No, the solutions have to be found in the music itself – in its rhythms, its dynamic shapes, the interaction of solo and mass forces. My present problem is that Ferneyhough seems to do everything at once and very fast. 'Seid umschlungen, Millionen' might well, in 'Carceri d'Invenzione', refer to the avalanche of notes and to the instructions for each of those notes.

Still, the challenge of putting the music of our own times on the television screen consists of finding a solution to one problem (of course, only to find that one solution has revealed another hundred problems). The relay of a concert is in many ways the least helpful way forward. Tele-vision anywhere has certain distinct duties of a public service kind, and in music that can mean bringing concerts to people and areas cut off from normal concert-going. However, the unadorned performance of new music may leave the television audience in a state of bewilderment and alienation. 'If that's new music, I'll stick with Brahms or Rachmaninov (or whoever), thanks all the same.' Even those involved in the transmission of new music can be similarly bemused. I remember a cameraman coming to me after the performance of a new work at the Proms and asking me very politely if I had been ordered to do it or whether I had volunteered. His astonishment was total, when I said that I had asked specially to direct the piece.

If television has a significant role to play in bringing together contemporary music and audiences (who are after all always contemporary), then it is not, I believe, in and from the concert hall. Rather, it is in the bold and continuous use of the medium's documentary possibilities. Television must examine the major musical events of the century, and equally it must encourage the writing of music specifically for television. In both cases the processes of 'how', 'why', and 'where' can be observed, recorded, and analysed. In fact, music documentaries occupy only the last 25 years of the medium's history. Ken Russell's brilliantly idiosyncratic fantasies on Elgar, Debussy, Prokofiev, and Bartok all date from the early 1960s. They were and remain a law unto themselves, responsible for outraging the music critics, who always know what you must not do, but responsible also for firing the enthusiasm of large audiences ready to learn and to be excited.

It was the advent of BBC 2 which made the music documentary a regular part of the television repertoire. It was Humphrey Burton, heading the original Music Department, who sensed the possibilities in both studio and film for giving a context to new music. I was fortunate to be in the right place at the right time. In fact, in 1964 I recall Humphrey collecting me one day and going down to the Maida Vale Studios to see a French composer conducting the BBC Symphony Orchestra. It was, of course, Pierre Boulez. 'He might be interesting' had been Humphrey's comment beforehand. In case that remark sounds inadequate, it should be remembered that Boulez was not then the world figure of today and anyway the spirit of both curiosity and adventure implicit in the comment were crucial to the development of a new kind of television music.

My collaboration with Boulez began that day in Maida Vale and has continued to the present. I have learnt from every minute of it, though I doubt very much whether there was anything for him to learn from television! Already in the mid-60s Boulez was preoccupied with the importance of marking out the major developments in twentieth-century music. Unlike many musicians, he has a highly developed visual sense, an encyclopaedic knowledge of the pictorial arts, and the ability to trace the ever closer connections between the different arts over the last 70 years. So in the late 60s and early 70s we made a number of films. The subject matter offers no great surprises – the Second Viennese School, the rhythmic inventions of Bartok and Stravinsky, outsiders like Ives and Varèse, Olivier Messiaen, Boulez's own music, and so on. However, we did try to break new ground in using metaphors from painting and architecture to make musical points. The programmes tended to be analytical in form and we used animated graphics to reveal the basic structures of the music. The performances were shot in ways that mirrored the musical construction – for example, the size of screen was changed, the editing was made more stylized and pronounced, and in short, we refused to hide behind the veneer of smooth, painless entertainment. Television technology has moved on a long way since then and in retrospect those early films seem laborious, over-busy, and rather mechanical. Still they did have something going for them.

Of course, it was not the only way forward. All too briefly around 1970 the BBC had on its staff a brilliant director from Australia, Bill Fitzwater. His style was free and radically innovative. His film on Harrison Birtwistle from that time should be seen again and his biography of Erik Satie still has the power to bowl me over with its exuberant, unbridled inventiveness. But the plain truth was that it takes more than one or two films a year, and more than one or two directors in an institution to build up a tradition of new music documentary.

The next head of BBC music was John Culshaw. He was basically hostile to all new music. Faced with a Boulez project he said on one

occasion: 'Oh! well, I suppose we have to do this kind of thing once in a while.' Not exactly a passionate commitment, and without that kind of commitment at a managerial level the basic inertia of institutional television towards new ideas and new risks takes control. In my view, the links between the medium and new music were stretched to breaking point. Certainly some films of quality were made, and in one case – Bryan Izzard's film of and about Berio's 'A-Ronne' – a film of quite remarkable brilliance appeared. However, to those of us who wanted to explore the television possibilities for contemporary music, the period from 1975 to 1985 was fairly arid. There is little more dispiriting than the experience of trying to make films for people who do not want them and who scarcely seem to notice their existence when you have made them.

Happily, changes are under way. The arrival of Channel 4 gave, at least at the outset, a new impetus to experiment. The 'Sinfonietta' series with Paul Crossley has been a significant success and marks a genuine return to the detailed examination and placing of music within the culture of this century. In the hands of five very different directors the series has examined not just the 'how' of major masterpieces from the last seven decades, but also the vital questions of 'why' and 'where'. The arrival of a vigorous new leadership in the BBC Music & Arts Department has opened up a whole new range of possibilities. Alan Yentob has committed himself to experiment and to adventure, no surprise perhaps from the former editor of 'Arena'. In appointing Dennis Marks to be in charge of music documentaries he has taken the first major step to make that commitment tangible. Once again, after a long hibernation, things are stirring. The phenomenon of Simon Rattle is crucial to the new activity. At last we have a world-class conductor with his own orchestra, who is not only ready to follow his own broad tastes in music of our time, but who is also an absolutely natural communicator both off and on the podium. Equally important, Rattle is unwilling to settle for the soft option of well-upholstered concert performances. Nor does he have any time for the 'personality profile' approach. It is precisely the documentary possibilities of music on television which attracts him. And, with no trace of arrogance, he knows his power. He can get Henze's Seventh Symphony or Berio's Sinfonia onto BBC 2; he can get Schoenberg and Robin Holloway onto Central TV.

Alongside this revival of basic music documentary, there is another prospect, at the moment less tangible and more notional. That is the examination of new music by making it specifically for television. There are plans within the BBC and Channel 4, plans which will involve the commissioning of pieces from contemporary composers. These would be pieces with a specific televisual component (though they could also exist in conventional concert form), and they would be framed within documentary material describing how they are created. By chance I am involved in a project which could be a pilot for future experiments – or perhaps just an awful warning! The composer Edward Cowie and I are making a film about Leonardo da Vinci. He has written a piece for small orchestra, suggesting possible images in the score, and I am working with Dave King, a film editor at the BBC of remarkable musicality, to realize these images on the screen. The result should be on BBC 2 early in 1987.

Like Lazarus, a bit the worse for wear but distinctly alive, the music documentary is back with us. Television policy has the habit of changing very quickly and it would be folly to be too sanguine. Nevertheless, the future for new music on the screen is potentially better than ever before. And by the way, how pleasant not to have to explain to one's superiors who George Benjamin is.

And now – back to Ferneyhough.

London's Other No. 10!

It is not too fanciful to call No. 10 Stratford Place, London W1, the 'new new music house'. There you will find many different musical organizations, the majority devoted solely to new music. The three with the most public face are the Society for the Promotion of New Music (SPNM), the Electro-Acoustic Music Association (EMAS), and the British Music Information Centre (BMIC).

SPNM promotes concerts and workshops featuring young and unknown composers' music. It also offers generous discounts on various new music products – for example records, tickets, and scores. SPNM also prepares the Contemporary Concerts Co-ordination brochure, an invaluable diary listing all the major twentieth-century music events in London and a selection from around the country. EMAS promotes interest in electro-acoustic music through its concerts and practical help with the loan of equipment and the provision of a general advisory service.

The British Music Information Centre is a reference library of British twentieth-century music, housing scores and recordings which amount to the largest collection of modern British music in the world. The library is free to use and there is no membership requirement and no appointment system. Twice a week, it becomes an evening concert venue for anyone to book for the presentation of predominately British twentieth-century music. A first come first served 'open door' policy has prevailed in the presentation of these events and the ensuing variety prevents any single artistic credo dominating the stage. In the following articles the work of the SPNM and EMAS are further described and the fascinating variety of BMIC events is listed.

Society for the Promotion of New Music
Rosemary Johnson, Administrator

A perennial subject of discussion at SPNM meetings is the level at which support should be given to young composers; whether or not it features on the agenda, it creeps in and opinion is always divided. There are protagonists for high-profile concerts which attract media attention to the Society and which give an undeniable fillip to a young composer's career with the possibilities of a BBC relay and good reviews in the national press, and there are those who support the salon event – small-scale, low-budget workshops, attended by the composer and few interested members of the general public (but definitely no press!) – where discussion is informal and mistakes can be made without losing face. The flip side of both approaches is all too obvious – media criticism is often harsh and if a young composer is not ready for public exposure it can be extraordinarily damaging, whereas with the small-scale workshop events, because of the greater number of works selected, artistic standards by necessity decline, and with them the reputation of the Society. The current SPNM Executive, with characteristic diplomacy, has tried to combine the best of both these worlds: over fifty pieces were selected for performance by the reading panel in the 12-month period between September 1985 and August 1986 (a significant increase on past statistics) ranging from enormous orchestral forces in the Barbican Hall to solo workshops in the more intimate setting of the BMIC. Geographically too, SPNM events were diverse, taking place as far afield as Southampton and Edinburgh, with additional festival appearances in Huddersfield, York, Brighton, and Bath. The main focus of London events became a newly-established monthly series of workshops and informal concerts at the BMIC housed, like the SPNM, at 10 Stratford Place.

The workshop process was repeated in more depth at the Annual Composers' Forum, which in 1985 was part of the first ever Southampton International Festival of New Music. In what was probably the only consistently fine week of the Summer the SPNM decamped to Southampton University where Gregory Rose's ensemble, Circle, provided a rival attraction to afternoon sunbathing, with energetic playing and constructive discussion on SPNM pieces, which varied in style from James Harley's elusive *Prelude* based on Japanese poems of Taeko Takaoni, to Richard Knight's jazz-inspired *Bongobebopoly*. In the morning the featured Festival composers, Hans Werner Henze, Alexander Goehr, and Simon Bainbridge gave seminars, in which they discussed their own music and listened to pieces by students at the Forum. Evening concerts were given by the Bournemouth Symphony Orchestra and Sinfonietta, the Arditti String Quartet, and the BBC Singers, of which the highlight was perhaps the towering performance of Henze's *Tristan* given by the BSO conducted by Oliver Knussen. Veterans of SPNM events were probably grateful that the week was not as frenetic as the 1985 Musica Nova Festival, but absent from Southampton was a central socializing/eating area with long licensing hours where informal discussion could continue.

At the extreme opposite of the spectrum were the two orchestral concerts promoted with very generous funding from the RVW Trust – one in the Philharmonic Hall, Liverpool and one in the Barbican Centre, London. Unperformed pieces were solicited more than a year in advance from composers over 25 and the 100 scores which arrived in the SPNM office were proof enough of the lack of opportunities available for composers who want the challenge of writing for a symphony orchestra. After much deliberation the reading panel – composers Alexander Goehr and Anthony Gilbert, conductor Elgar Howarth, and Bernard Benoliel, administrator of the RVW Trust – selected four of the scores: Glynn Perrin's *Tu, même*, Steve Martland's *Babi Yar*, Silvina Milstein's *Sombras*, and Michael Rosenzweig's *Symphony in one movement*. The length of the resulting programme would have taxed the endurance of even the most avid contemporary music fan, and created a rehearsal schedule of gargantuan proportions, so it was decided to include the Milstein piece, the smallest in scale, in another SPNM concert scheduled later in the year. This left us with Perrin,

Rosenzweig, and Martland, whose photographs, at least for the two weeks preceding the concert, leapt out of the pages of every publication with even a remote musical interest. Sadly the project proved too ambitious to accomplish in the time available, even despite the generous rehearsal allocation: Glynn Perrin's extraordinary complex piece, written as part of his doctorate for York University and far removed from his current work with the band Man Jumping, was the casualty. In Liverpool a play-through of one section was attempted but in the end it seemed more rewarding to concentrate on the other two pieces to provide a more happily structured evening. *Babi Yar*, inspired by Anatoli Kuznetsov's book which details the slaughter of 200,000 civilians, most of them Jews, by the Nazis and Russians during the Second World War, is a powerful, battering piece which divides the orchestra into three separate performing groups and adds to the normal orchestral complement electric guitar, bass guitar, three saxophones, and Hammond organ. Rosenzweig's *Symphony in one movement*, with its sextet of flutes and extensive percussion section, is in contrast far more lyrical and reflective. Although the Society very much regrets that *Tu, même* was not performed on this occasion, the RLPO have undertaken to include the piece in their future schedule with a substantial allocation of rehearsal time. Debate about whether the three pieces should have been programmed into one concert or spread through the course of a season is inevitable given the circumstances, but the Society is only too aware that its normal funding makes no provision for the performance of works for such large forces and is more than grateful to the RVW Trust for making the project possible.

Two happy firsts of the year were coincidentally both workshop events; one in association with Arnolfini in Bristol and the second a collaboration with the York Spring Festival of Contemporary Music. In Bristol Uroboros spent an intensive day on five pieces which included two minimalist works: David Morris's *Anton Bruckner meets Steve Reich* and Glenn Sweet's *Aria of the Grand Duke* (which turned out to be twice as long as the composer's original estimate of 14 minutes, and reminded us how important it is for composers to calculate an accurate duration!). The cosy atmosphere of Arnolfini lent itself extremely well to this kind of discussion event and it is very much hoped that the Society will return there in the near future. At York, Harrison Birtwistle, who with Peter Maxwell Davies has very recently become a vice president of the SPNM, spent the morning listening to performances of five works (three selected by the Society) and the afternoon discussing compositional points with the composers and the considerable audience who had turned up to listen and indeed participate. The Society is delighted to welcome our new vice-presidents and hope that this type of practical involvement will continue.

The season finished on a high. Through another vice-president, Alexander Goehr, the Society was invited to take part in the Edinburgh Festival in a weekend of contemporary music personally devised by Goehr and featuring twentieth-century classics as well as a number of premières. Philip Cashian's *Moon of the Dawn* was exquisitely sung by the young soprano Carol Smith with fine playing from the Brodsky String Quartet. The whole programme, which included works by Stravinsky, Lutoslawski, and Bartok was recorded by the BBC for later relay.

So, what lies in the future for the SPNM? Debate will still continue on the subject of high-profile concerts versus workshops, and there has also been serious discussion about the reading panel process and the planning of concerts. Comment from the Society's members is always very welcome and, by the way, membership is not exclusive to composers. Membership is open to anyone interested in contemporary music and members enjoy a wide range of benefits. Our mail order service for opera tickets, records, scores, and books on contemporary music has continued to grow in the past year and is particularly appreciated by those outside London for whom many of these items are hard to find. Membership subscriptions are a very vital part of our income and make a significant contribution towards helping promote our SPNM concerts.

The success of all SPNM events ultimately depends on the calibre of the scores received by the reading panel. We are anxious to find as great a range of styles and pieces as possible and hope this year to encourage a number of new composers to submit their work. There are no limits on instrumentation, and tape pieces and works with electronic treatment are also welcome. Composers must be British or resident in the UK, but there are no age limits imposed. Should you wish to find out about sending scores to the SPNM or more about membership please do write or drop in to 10 Stratford Place, London W1N 9AE, telephone 01-491 8111.

Report of events September 1985 to August 1986

September 9–13 Southampton University 19th Annual Composers' Forum. 4 days of workshops given by Circle directed by Gregory Rose on pieces by Charles Barber, Robin Gosnall, Robin Grant, James Harley, Lawrence Hughes, Robert Keeley, Richard Knight, and Peter Seabourne. Seminar on Notation led by David Bedford and Colin Matthews. Part of the Southampton International Festival of New Music.

November 19–20 Huddersfield Festival Workshops and Concert. Two workshops on aspects of playing contemporary brass music given by Equale Brass and a final concert which included the première of a work by Philip Feeney.

November 22 Philharmonic Hall, Liverpool RVW Trust Concert. World premières for orchestral works by Steve Martland and Michael Rosenzweig given by the Royal Liverpool Philharmonic Orchestra under Nicholas Cleobury.

November 25 Barbican Centre, London RVW Trust Concert. Repeat of November 22 performance.

December 10 EMI Studios, Abbey Road Open Orchestral Rehearsal. The London Sinfonietta and Rosemary Hardy under Oliver Knussen presented an open rehearsal on works by Nicholas Harberd and David Sawer.

January 31 St John's, Smith Square
Orchestral Concert. The National Centre for
Orchestral Studies Symphony Orchestra under
Adrian Leaper performed orchestral works by
Martin Butler, Colin Griffith, and Silvina Milstein.

February 17 The Place, Camden
Chamber Concert. Exposé performed works by
Charles Barber, James Clarke, Stanley Haynes, and
David Lancaster.

March 10 The Place, Camden
Chamber Concert. Phoenix Wind Quintet
performed works by Robin Gosnall and Ho Wai On.

March 12 Guildhall School of Music
Chamber Concert. 20th Century Music Enterprise
performed a work by David Lancaster.

March 13 Guildhall School of Music
Recital. Roger Heaton performed a new work by
John Wilks.

March 15 Arnolfini, Bristol
Workshop. Uroboros under Gwyn Pritchard gave
a workshop on pieces by Richard Knight, David
Morris, Peter Seabourne, Glenn Sweet, and Param
Vir. Workshop Director, David Bedford.

March 20 York University
Workshop. Students of the University gave
workshop performances of pieces by James Erber,
Phillip Harris, and Malcolm Hayes under the
direction of Harrison Birtwistle. Part of the York
Spring Festival.

April 16 St John's, Smith Square
Concert. Uroboros under Gwyn Pritchard gave

the first performance of Param Vir's piece selected
from the Bristol workshop on March 15.

May 12 BMIC
Workshop. Michael Finnissy talked about and
performed works by David Aldridge, Christopher
Best, Philip Cashian, and Peter Graham.

May 21 The Music Room, Brighton
Concert. The first performance of work by Erika
Fox given by Lontano under Odaline de la
Martinez. Part of the Brighton Festival.

May 30 Guildhall, Bath
Concert. Music Projects/London under Richard
Bernas gave performances of works by Javier
Alvarez, Paul Archbold, and James Clarke. Part of
the Bath Festival.

June 11 Almeida Theatre, London
Concert. Capricorn under Grant Llewellyn
performed works by Rupert Bawden, James Dillon,
and Simon Holt.

June 16 BMIC
Workshop. Workshop performances of pieces by
John Michael Clarke, Richard Dinnadge, and
Michael Rosas Cobian given by the Fairfield
Quartet under the direction of Justin Connolly.

July 3 BMIC
Informal Concert. Pieces by Javier Alvarez, Paul
Archbold, Philip Feeney, and Robin Walker
performed by Mandala.

August 23 Queen's Hall, Edinburgh
Concert. First performance of a piece by Philip
Cashian given by the Brodsky Quartet and Carol
Smith. Part of the Edinburgh Festival.

Electro-Acoustic Music Association
Simon Emmerson, Chairperson

The Electro-Acoustic Music Association of Great
Britain was founded in January 1979 with the
intention of promoting all aspects of this unique
development in twentieth-century music. From
the outset membership was intended to include not
only composers and performers but also publishers, studios, manufacturers, and any interested
laypeople. EMAS has continued to expand from its
initial 100 members to a figure at least three times
that with a substantial overseas membership. In
1984, following 5 years in which the organization
was run entirely by volunteers, EMAS gained a
grant from the Arts Council for the appointment of
an administrator for an initial 2-year period, now
renewed for a further 2 years. The next stage of

EMAS' development will be a drive to raise
sponsorship for some aspects of its work. Concert
promotion, educational activities, and courses are
planned to increase still further the very substantial amount that EMAS already does with its
restricted resources.

One of the most important channels of
information which EMAS has established is the
first journal – called simply 'Electroacoustic
Music' – to cover this area (notwithstanding the
many journals available for the more popular
music applications). The journal is truly national,
being edited, assembled, and distributed in Birmingham and Newcastle. It aims to cover technical,
aesthetic, and musical issues as well as covering
general news items from members, studios, etc. An
important offshoot of the journal has been the bi-
monthly Concert Agenda which aims to list as
many concerts, events, conferences, prizes, etc, as
possible, which involve electroacoustic elements.

EMAS also runs a mailout service which allows concert promoters and publishers to target its specific interests.

The EMAS international concert series is now in its fourth year. The aims have been broad. It is a monthly concert series which acts as a regular forum for new works from Britain and abroad. Although resources have limited the live performance element in the series a huge variety of new works has been premièred (or, just as importantly, given second performances) in Britain. In addition, a series of collaborations have been staged with bodies such as the Society for the Promotion of New Music, the Almeida Festival, the American Festival, the Dartington Summer School, and various individual ensembles. These have enabled far more ambitious projects to be mounted, including weekend seminars and concerts, and the complete 'backup' for the 'Steve Reich at Fifty' concerts at the Almeida Festival '86. EMAS plans to expand much more into the regions in future years. Already concerts have been presented in Southampton, Liverpool, and Dartington, and assistance given to many organizations throughout the country.

Shortly after its foundation, EMAS gained a substantial equipment grant from the Arts Council to establish a store of quality concert equipment, for both its own use and to hire to others. This has allowed EMAS not only to run its own concert series but also to develop links with major performance organizations throughout the country. While the income generated is not substantial, it has allowed the updating and expansion of this resource.

Educational projects have been organized in many schools and colleges. This aspect of EMAS' activities is being actively encouraged in a drive to gain support for sponsorship and equipment. Concert/workshops, talks, and demonstrations are available for teachers, students, and clubs. EMAS members in the regions are being encouraged to organize locally with the support of the London office. Demonstrations of both equipment and techniques of composition are planned.

As an advice centre, EMAS receives dozens of phone calls asking for help on everything from school projects to concert presentation, and this puts an enormous responsibility on the single administrator. In future EMAS plans to automate some of the more laborious parts of this work, creating a series of information sheets. We do not confine our advice to members, but try to persuade the non-members among those who contact us that it would be well worth joining!

Membership services are being developed slowly. Since the earliest days, studio members have organized Technical Seminars aimed at getting specific problems discussed. Topics are defined by the host studio and may vary from computer applications to problems such as exchanging tapes and standardizing formats. Individual members are invited and the number participating has been high. A report usually appears in the journal.

One of EMAS' most important roles lies in the international field. The existence of a national organization allows effective exchange and a more extensive liaison with organizations overseas. Recently EMAS has had contact with IRCAM (Paris), MIT (Cambridge, Mass.), Stanford (California), EMS (Stockholm), and many other smaller groups. Tapes and other concert materials are exchanged, composers visit, and valuable contacts are made. EMAS is a member of the ICEM (International Confederation for Electroacoustic Music) with by far the largest public membership of the affiliated organizations. Indeed EMAS was the first such organization in the world and is the model for several others which have been founded subsequently.

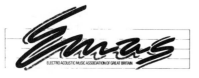

ELECTRO-ACOUSTIC MUSIC ASSOCIATION OF GREAT BRITAIN

the national organisation promoting the aims of research, composition and performance in the field of electro-acoustic music.

Electro-acoustic music covers all types of music requiring electronic technology, from musique concrète and electronic music, to live electronics, computers and microprocessors. EMAS publishes a quarterly newsletter, organises meetings and technical seminars, runs a monthly concert series and administers a Sound Equipment Pool of high quality for concert playback. The concert series features international soloists, dance, and new works for multimedia, live-electronics and tape.

Membership is open to musicians, dancers, visual artists, and anyone else with an interest in electronic music.

For information and details of membership, contact:

**10 Stratford Place
London W1N 9AE
Telephone 01-499 2576**

EMAS also campaigns for the establishment of a national studio for electroacoustic composition and a properly equipped performance space for the music. Existing studios in Britain are restricted in access (usually being in universities) and are in need of substantial upgrading in many respects. EMAS has been active in recent discussions to establish a national studio, not so much along the lines of the large centralized studios of the 60s and 70s, but instead considering the possibilities of developing a centre from which a national software network could be developed to assist home composition. The central studio would be needed only for specialist applications not yet available on home computers. The provision of a fully equipped performance space, especially one purpose built, is more difficult to foresee. Perhaps even part of a disused warehouse would do if a sponsor could be found!

EMAS hopes to celebrate its 10th birthday in style with a major international festival. Let us hope that it marks the coming age of electroacoustic music.

Report of Events
September 1985 to August 1986

☆☆☆ First performance
☆☆ First British performance
☆ First London performance

October 26
St John's, Smith Square
A 50th Birthday Concert for Barry Anderson
Barry Anderson *Fanfare; Colla Voce*
Karlheinz Stockhausen *Solo*
Barry Anderson *Piano Pieces 2 and 3; Mask* ☆☆☆

Jane Manning (sop), Kathryn Lukas (fl), Sally Mays (pno), Simon Limbrick (perc), Peter Harlowe (narrator), The West Square Electronic Music Ensemble (director Barry Anderson), Javier Alvarez and Stephen Montague (sound projection)

A series of three concerts given by the Arditti Quartet with Stephen Montague (sound projection) at the Almeida Theatre. The Quartet used a quartet of electrically-based strings conceived and developed in Canada by Raad Instruments (works denoted by ●).

November 3
Brian Ferneyhough *String Quartet No. 2*
Bengt Sorenson *Alman* ☆☆
Chris Dench *Strangeness* ☆☆
Roger Redgate *Quartet No. 2* ☆☆
Michael Nyman *Quartet* ●

November 10
Jurg Wittenbach *Execution ajournée 2*
Sven-David Sandström *Behind* ☆☆

Gavin Bryars *Quartet* ● ☆☆☆
Roger Reynolds *'Coconino . . . a shattered landscape'* ☆☆☆

November 17
Klaus Hubler *Musica Mensurabilis (Quartet No. 3)* ☆☆
Karl Rasmussen *Surrounded by Scales* ☆☆
Gilberto Cappelli *Quartet No. 1* ☆☆
Volker Heyn *Sirenes* ☆
Tim Souster *Quartet with tape* ● ☆☆☆

December 2
The Place Theatre
Dennis Smalley *Pentes*
Bernard Parmegiani *De Natura Sonorum*

Jonty Harrison (sound projection)

January 15
City University
Meet the Composer; Gerald Shapiro

January 20
The Place Theatre
Daniel Lentz *King Speech Song* ☆☆
Otto Luening *Low Speed*
Wlodzimierz Kotonski *Etude on a Single Cymbal Stroke* ☆☆
Simon Emmerson *Recollections* ☆☆☆
Rolf Enström *Final Curses* ☆☆
Alan Belk *One Man Show* ☆☆☆

Alan Belk (voice), Simon Emmerson, Javier Alvarez, and Stephen Montague (sound projection)

January 30
Morley College
Meet the Composer; Jonathan Kramer

February 25
City University
Meet the Composer; Roger Smalley
Roger Smalley *Pulses; Echo III*
Giacinto Scelsi *I Presaggi* ☆☆☆

Music Projects/London, Richard Bernas (director)
Simon Emmerson and Roger Smalley (sound projection)

March 6
Morley College
Meet the Composer; Ron Perera

March 13
The Place Theatre
Meet the Composer: Denis Lorrain
Richard Zvonar *3 for 5* ☆☆
Simon Limbrick/Ian Spink *One Small Step*
Denis Lorrain *The Other Shape* ☆☆
Frederic Rzewski *Lost and Found*

Simon Limbrick (perc), Denis Lorrain and Stephen Montague (sound projection)

March 14 and 15
The Place Theatre
Two evenings of dance with four young choreographers
Celia Hutton, music by Denis Smalley

Pablo Ventura, music by Reed Holmes
Darshan Bhuller, music by Barry Guy
Jonathan Lunn, music by Schoenberg

April 23
The Place Theatre
Bernard Parmegiani *Dedans Dehors*
Simon Emmerson *Windbreak* ☆
Michael McNabb *Dreamsong*
Alejandro Viñao *Go*

John Wallace (tpt), Simon Emmerson (sound projection)

May 25
Almeida Theatre
Michael Gordon *Acid Rain* ☆☆
James Sellars *Return of the Comet* ☆☆
Jonathan Kramer *Renaissance* ☆☆
Michael Torke *Vanada* ☆☆

Spectrum, Guy Protheroe (director), Javier Alvarez and Stephen Montague (sound projection)

June 20
Almeida Theatre
New works for shakuhachi and tape by Richard Attree, Ian Dearden, Andrew Lewis, Michael Turnbull, and Michael Vaughan

Yashikazu Iwamoto (shakuhachi)

June 28 and 29
Almeida Festival, Almeida Theatre and Union Chapel
A Steve Reich Weekend
Circle, director Gregory Rose, Steve Reich (sound projection)

British Music Information Centre
Roger Wright

Concert Listings, September 1985 to September 1986

☆☆☆ First performance
☆☆ First British performance
☆ First London performance

September 17
Anthony Gilbert *Piano Sonata No. 1*
Ferrucio Busoni *Sonatina No. 4*
Laurence Crane *Preludes 6–8* ☆☆☆
Robert Keeley *From Ground to Air* ☆☆☆
J. S. Bach *Two Preludes and Fugues*
Olivier Messiaen *Le Traquet Rieur*

Robert Keeley (pno)

September 19
Pawlu Grech *Quaderno II; Duo I; Five Events*
Messiaen *Quatuor pour la fin du temps*

Clare Thompson (vln), Justin Pearson (vc), Philip Edwards (cl), David Elwin (pno)

September 26
Malcolm Dedman *Metamorphoses on the raga Puria Dahaneshri; Meditation No. 2*
Dorothy Strutt *Through a glass darkly*
Martin Vishnick *Meditation*

Malcolm Dedman (synthesizer, keybd, crotales), Janet Dedman (pno), Dorothy Strutt (pno, keybd, vc), Martin Vishnick (electric guitar)

October 3
Kenneth V. Jones *Dialysis*
Carl Rutti *The Secret Rose*
Timothy Higgs *Sonata in D*
Neil Saunders *Three Songs of Innocence*
David Gow *Scorpio*

Petronella Dittmer (vln), Richard Coulson (hpschd)

October 8
Buxton Orr *Bagatelles*
Peter Carr *Short Sonata No. 3*
Carey Blyton *Carp in the Rain*
Eric Hudes *Fantasia (quasi una sonata)*

Malcolm Dedman *Spectrum*
Bernard Stevens *Ballad No. 2*
Timothy Moore *Prelude and Fugue in C*
Frank Bayford *Autumn Changes*
Michael Maxwell *Two Inventions* ☆
Hugh Wood *Three Piano Pieces Op. 5*
John Mitchell *Three Pieces for vibraphone*

Derek Foster (pno and vibraphone)

October 10
Patrick Morris *Scherzino; Romance; Prelude;
    Lament; Lorelei; Devotion; A Post-Industrial
    Melody*
Laurence Crane *Preludes 1–8*
Howard Skempton *Slow Waltz; Twin Set; Deeply
    Shaded; Wedding Tune; Small Change; Home
    and Abroad; Recessional*

The Wink: Ian Wilson (fl), Nicolas Cherniavski
(vc), Laurence Crane (pno and perc), Patrick
Morris (pno) with Howard Skempton (accordion)

October 14
William Hurlstone *Sonata in F major*
Patric Standford *Four Preludes*
Elizabeth Maconchy *Concertino (2nd and 3rd
    movts)*
Marcus Blunt *Caprice and Scotch Song* ☆☆☆
Edward Elgar *Romance*
Roger Steptoe *Two Studies* ☆
Gilbert Vinter *The Playful Pachyderm*

Jean Owen (bn), Hilary Punshon (pno)

October 17
Lennox Berkeley *Sonata; Sonatina*
Michael Regan *Two Pieces*
Arthur Honegger *Danse de la chèvre*
Paul Hindemith *Sonata*
Claude Debussy *Syrinx*
Giulio Briccialdi *Carnival of Venice Op. 78*

Adrian Spence (fl), Jane Compton (pno)

October 22
Eugene Goossens *Kaleidoscope*
Percy Grainger *To a Nordic Princess; Irish Tune
    from County Derry; Country Gardens*
Stephen Windos/Bennett Hogg *Improvisation*

Stephen Windos (pno)

October 24
Edward Watson *Three Shakespeare Songs* ☆
Derek Foster *Andante*
Sydney Vale *Barque of Phosphor*
Constance Warren *Cradle Song* ☆
John Mitchell *Three Housman Songs*
Marcus Blunt *Venus Eclipsed*
Arnold Cooke *Three Songs of Innocence*
Peter Collins *Three Songs of Innocence* ☆
Herbert Howells *Sonata for clarinet and piano*
John McCabe *Three Folksongs*

Microcosmos: Pauline Alder (sop), Peter Gosling
(cl), John Gough (pno)

October 30
Charles Ives *Violin Sonata No. 2*
Virgil Thomson *Serenade for flute and violin*
Peter Maxwell Davies *Solita; Hill Runes*
Arthur Berger *Trio for violin, guitar, and piano*
Helen Roe *Verbum supernum prodiens/Conditor
    alme siderum*
Robert Sherlaw Johnson *Projections* ☆

Mandala (fl, vln/vla, guitar, and pno)

November 5
Lennox Berkeley *Three Greek Songs*
Alan Bullard *Two Songs (The Shepherd to his
    love/The year's awakening)*
Stuart Scott *Songs of the Night* ☆☆☆
Michael Head *Three Songs of Venice*
Eric Hudes *Sapho Fragments*
Ernest Baker *Two Poems of Rostrevor Hamilton*
Anthony Campbell Allen *One Song from 'Another
    Spring'*
Antony Elton *Two Shakespeare Songs*
Geoffrey Bush *Three Songs (Rutterkin, When May
    is his prime, and Carol)*

Vanessa Smith (sop), Roger Crocker (pno)

November 7
Cornelius Cardew *Charge!; Bring the land a new
    life; Soon; Long live Chairman Mao!; The
    Croppy Boy; Song and Dance*
Jo Kondo *Walk*
Michael Parkin *Elegy*
Lennox Berkeley *Sonatina*
J. B. Priest *'Trotz der verspätung sind wir bereit'*
Kazuo Fukushima *Three Pieces from Chu-u*
Arghyris Kounadis *Blues*

Nancy Ruffer (fl), Walter Fabeck (pno)

November 11
York Bowen *Suite No. 2*
Alan Rawsthorne *The Creel*
Claude Debussy *Six Epigraphes Antiques*
Constant Lambert *Trois Pièces Nègres*
Igor Stravinsky *The Rite of Spring*

Kathryn Page and John Lenehan (pno duet)

November 12
Benjamin Dale *Fantasy Op. 4; Romance (from
    Suite Op. 2); Introduction and Allegro*
Constance Warren *Four Pieces for piano* ☆
Julius Harrison *Sonata in C minor*

Terence Nettle, Bridget Carey, Rachel Bolt,
Matthew Fairman, Christopher Yates, Katherine
Leek (vlas), Michael Jones (pno)

November 14
Leo Brouwer *Three Pieces*
Colin Downs *Mosaic*
Reginald Smith Brindle *Sonata No. 4*
John Duarte *Idylle pour Ida*
Pujol *Three Pieces*
Ray Burley (guitar)

November 19

Jacques Ibert *Entracte*
Edward Cowie *Mount Keira Duets* ☆☆
Melvyn Cann *Music for Healing*
Jonathan Lloyd *Suite: The Five Senses* ☆☆
Mario Castelnuovo-Tedesco *Sonatina Op. 205*
Francis Routh *Dance Interludes Op. 47* ☆☆
Alison Bauld *Monody for flute*
David Bedford *You asked for it*
Heitor Villa-Lobos *Distribucao des flores;
    Bachianas Brasileiras No. 5 (Cantilena); Prelude
    No. 4; Flute Flight (arr. Walker)*

Judith Hall (fl), Timothy Walker (guitar)

November 27

Frederick Delius *Irmelin; In the garden of the
    seraglio; La lune blanche; Avant que tu ne t'en
    ailles; Two Interludes (arr. Fenby); Nach neuen
    Meeren; Der Wandrer und sein Schatten;
    Twilight Fancies; Hidden Love; So white, so soft,
    so sweet is she; The Page; The Nightingale;
    Sehnsucht; Young Venevil; The Homeward Way;
    Love's Philosophy*
Ralph Vaughan Williams *Blake Songs*
John Ireland *Ragamuffin; Soliloquy; Merry Andrew*
Benjamin Britten *Pan/Phaeton/Arethusa (from Six
    Metamorphoses after Ovid)*
York Bowen *Oboe Sonata*

Rachel Sherry (sop), Margaret Roberts (pno),
Victoria Trotman (ob)

November 28

Dorothea Franchi *Mädchensliebe* ☆☆
Edmund Rubbra *Two Songs for voice and harp*
Sydney Vale *Three of Four Hills and a Cloud* ☆☆☆;
    *Bagatelle; The Grey Spires of
    Dawn* ☆☆☆;*Toccata Humoresque*
Derek Foster *Study for solo vibraphone* ☆☆☆
Alan Bullard *Variations on an English Folk Tune*
Joyce Barrell *Partita for solo vibraphone* ☆
Frank Bayford *Piano Sonata No. 1*
William Wordsworth *Valediction*
Frank Bayford *Stanford Bagatelles* ☆☆☆
Marcus Blunt *Iona Prelude and Caprice*

Lilian Newman (sop), David Snell (hp), Derek
Foster (vibraphone and pno), John Mitchel (pno)

December 5

Howard Skempton *Quavers 3; Simple Piano Piece;
    Gentle Melody; Spring Waltz; merry-go-round;
    Christmas Melody; Twin Set, and Pearls*
Patrick Morris *Prelude; Lament; Profound
    Nostalgia; Aspirations; Moonscape; Salamander*
Laurence Crane *Preludes 6–8; Three Melodies*

The Wink; Ian Wilson (fl), Nicolas Cherniavski
(vc), Laurence Crane (pno and perc), Patrick
Morris (pno) with Howard Skempton and John
Chilton (accordions)

December 6

Peter Dickinson *An e e cummings song cycle;
    Piano Transformations; Stevie's Tunes; An
    anthology; Piano Pieces; Extravaganzas; Song:
    So we'll go no more a-roving; Schubert in Blue*

Meriel Dickinson (mezzo-sop), Peter Dickinson
(pno)

December 9

Jonathan Harvey *Transformations*
Judith Weir *Sketches from a Bagpiper's Album*
Jonathan Lloyd *True Refuge* ☆
Hugh Wood *Paraphrase*
York Bowen *Clarinet Sonata*

Nicholas Cox (cl), Vanessa Latarche (pno)

December 10

Martyn Harry *Ozymandias for cello and piano* ☆
Phanos Dymiotis *Duo for violin and piano* ☆
Matthew Taylor *String Quartet No. 2* ☆
David Lancaster *Two pieces for oboe and
    piano* ☆☆☆

Phanos Dymiotis, Colin Huehns (vlns), Nick Booth
(vla), Cathy Durham (vc), Ruth Watson (ob),
David Aldridge, Alan Mills, Murray McLachlan
(pno)

December 12

Kenneth V. Jones *Violin Sonata*
Frank Stiles *Sonata for solo violin*
Bernard Stevens *Violin Sonata*
David Nevens *Piano Work* ☆
John Kinsella *Rhapsody on a poem by Joseph
    Campbell*
Thomas Wilson *Violin Sonata*
David Harries *Six Impromptus*

Clarence Myerscough (vln), Geoffrey Buckley
(pno)

December 17

Lord Berners *Dispute entre le papillon et le crapaud*
Peter Warlock *Folk Song Preludes Nos. 2 and 3*
Percy Grainger *One more day, my John*
Bernard Stevens *Fuga alla sarabanda* ☆☆☆
Michael Finnissy *GFH* ☆☆☆
Howard Skempton *Eirenicon 4* ☆☆☆
Chris Newman *Nice Nights/nette Nächte/Les Nuits
    gentille* ☆☆☆
Richard Barrett *heard* ☆☆☆
Judith Weir *Michael's Strathspey* ☆☆☆
Alan Bush *Mister Playford's Tunes*

Michael Finnissy (pno)

1986
January 7

Francis Poulenc *Flute Sonata*
Richard Rodney Bennett *Winter Music*
Oliver Knussen *Masks*
Rhián Samuel *Caprice* ☆☆☆
Luciano Berio *Sequenza 1*
Albert Roussel *Les joueurs de flûte*
Duncan Druce *Lacerta Agilis (Sand Lizard)*
Olivier Messiaen *Le merle noir*

Barbara Dolejal (fl), Esther Cavett-Dunsby (pno)

January 9
Paul Hancock *24 Preludes* ☆; *. . . in silence . . .* ☆; *6 Little piano pieces* ☆☆☆; *Maen tans – Boskednan* ☆

Paul Hancock (pno)

January 14
Ralph Vaughan Williams *Blake Songs*
Michael Tippett *Songs for Ariel*
George Messervy *Time Eating for tenor, oboe, and piano* ☆☆☆; *Exogen for solo oboe* ☆☆☆; *Time Path for solo piano* ☆
Elizabeth Routier *Songs from the cycle 'Not waving but Drowning'* ☆
Robert Saxton *Cantata No. 2*

Rogers Covey-Crump (tenor), Robin Canter (ob), Michael Freyhan (pno)

January 16
Paul Patterson *Comedy for five winds*
Elizabeth Maconchy *Wind Quintet*
Robin Holloway *Divertimento (Nursery Rhymes)*

Eileen Hulse (sop), Vanbrugh Wind Quintet

January 21
Gordon Jacob *Three Songs*
Ralph Vaughan Williams *Three Vocalises*
Peter Graham *Moments for piano* ☆☆
Matyas Seiber *Drei Morgenstern Lieder*
Michael Head *The Singer*
Franz Schubert *Das hirt auf dem Felsen*

Mary Porter (sop), Stephen Dehn (cl), Angela Hewitt (pno)

January 27
John White *Eight Waltzes from Basingstoke; Six Concert Duos*
Christopher Hobbs *Twelve Sketches for tuba and piano; Four Pieces for tuba and keyboards*

John White (tba and keybds), Christopher Hobbs (keybds)

January 30
Patric Standford *Variations*
John McCabe *Five Bagatelles*
William Lloyd Webber *Three Spring Miniatures*
Anthony Payne *Paean*
Martin Ellerby *Nocturnes* ☆
Puay Kiang Seng *Two Studies* ☆☆☆
Michael Regan *Five studies* ☆☆☆

Richard Deering (pno)

January 31
Priaulx Rainier *Pastoral Triptych; Barbaric Dance Suite; Suite for solo cello; Suite for clarinet and piano; The Bee Oracles (played on tape)*
Elisabeth Lutyens *Duo for oboe and violin*

Joyce Rathbone (pno), Joan Dickson (vc), Perry Hart (vln), George Caird (ob), Duncan Prescott (cl), Scott Mitchell (pno)

February 4
Ian Gardiner *Small World; Green Park* ☆☆☆;

Charing Cross ☆☆☆; *21st century foxtrot*
Andrew Thomson *The Gymnosophist* ☆☆☆; *Sabotherm; Simon and Ennoia*

George W. Welch Ensemble

February 6
Duncan Druce *Lacerta Agilis*
Jonathan Harvey *Nataraja* ☆
Ernest Baker *Night Theme*
Enid Luff *Canto and Doubles*
Patric Standford *Four Preludes*
Herbert Howells *Grace for a Fresh Egg*
Michael Norris *Pros and Cons*
Julia Usher *Aquarelles*
Frank Stiles *Keyboard Sonata*
Neil Sissons *Passacaglia*
Heitor Villa-Lobos *Bachianas Brasileiras No. 6*

Clive Conway (fls), Gwyn Parry-Jones (bn), Neil Sissons (pno)

February 7
Brian Dennis *The Recruiting Officer (from Night Cycle); Wandering Breezes; A Little Water Music; Songs of the Autumn Sunset; Three Poems of the Wang River*

Brian Dennis (bar), Peter Hill (pno)

February 11
Adrian Cruft *Stratford Music; Two Corantos; Three Miniatures; Concertante; Two English Keyboard Pieces; Three Bagatelles; Dance Movement*
All these pieces received two performances

New Wind Quintet, Alistair Young (pno)

February 13
Michael Finnissy *English Country-Tunes (revised version)* ☆☆☆

Michael Finnissy (pno)

February 18
Stephen Deutsch *Canons* ☆☆☆; *Attenuated Love Songs; Sextet* ☆☆☆; *Three Pieces for clarinet* ☆☆☆; *Superfluous Love Songs; Overtones*

Christine Page (sop), Pamela Lidiard (pno), David Campbell, Andrew Sparling (cls), Fairfield String Quartet

February 25
Michael Tippett *Piano Sonata No. 2*
Anton Webern *Five Canons*
Alexander Goehr *Prelude and Fugue*
Oliver Knussen *Trumpets*
William Walton *Three Sitwell Songs*
York Bowen *Clarinet Sonata*
Dominick Argento *To be sung upon the water*

Eileen Hulse (sop), Jeremy Rose, Ian Mitchell, Colin Honour (cls), Paul Turner (pno), Gregory Rose (director)

February 27
Harrison Birtwistle *Précis*
Peter Maxwell Davies *Five Little Pieces*

Alexander Goehr *Three Piano Pieces*
Thea Musgrave *Monologue*
Christopher Best *Piano Sonata –
    Reconciliations* ☆☆☆
Michael Tippett *Piano Sonata No. 1*
Pierre Boulez *Piano Sonata No. 3*

Raymond Clarke (pno)

March 3

Bernard Stevens *Fantasia on 'Giles Farnaby's
    Dreame'; Fantasia for two violins and piano;
    Nocturne on a note-row of Ronald Stevenson;
    Piano Sonata in one movement; Birthday Song;
    Fuga alla sarabanda*
Edwin Roxburgh *Etudes Nos. 3 and 5*
John White *Sonata No. 103*
Michael Finnissy *BS* ☆☆☆
Adrian Williams *Jubilypso*

Michael Finnissy, James Gibb (pnos), Sybil
Copeland, Jack Glickman (vlns), Isabel Beyer and
Harvey Dagul (pno duet)

March 4

Scott Willcox *No Blows were Struck; Three by Five*
Peter Anthony Monk *Appeelkins; Sonnet for solo
    clarinet; The Emperor's New Notes*
Julie Ainscough *Six poems of Emily Brontë*

Patricia Forbes (sop), Leon Ogden, Robert Millett,
Mary Keating (perc), Hiscock Brass, Kevin Hall,
Peter Heron (cls)

March 12

Alexander Goehr *Paraphrase on Monteverdi's 'Il
    Combattimento'*
Arnold Bax *Piano Sonata No. 2*
Paul Patterson *Conversations*
Alban Berg *Four Pieces*
Krzysztof Penderecki *Three Miniatures*
Max Reger *Sonata in A flat*

Duncan Prescott (cl), Scott Mitchell (pno)

March 18

Laurence Crane *10,000 Green Bottles; Preludes
    1–5; Air, Processional*
Howard Skempton *Third Suite; Something of an
    occasion; Small change, Axis, Air Melody*
Patrick Morris *Devotion, Cradle Song; In
    Memoriam, Adios, and Farewell; A Post-
    Industrial Melody, Solitude*

The Wink; Su Peasgood (fl), Alan Brett (vc),
Laurence Crane (pno and perc), Patrick Morris
(pno) with Howard Skempton (accordion)

March 19

Aaron Copland *Duo*
Robert Hinchliffe *The Elements*
Bohuslav Martinů *Scherzo*
Gavin Greenaway *Three canons* ☆☆☆
Albert Roussel *Joueurs de flûte*
Ralph Vaughan Williams *Suite de ballet*

Paul Raybould (fl), Gavin Greenaway (pno)

March 25

Sergei Rachmaninov *Two Preludes*
Eric Hudes *Fantasia (quasi una sonata)*
Claude Debussy *Estampes*
Jonathan Darnborough *Clowns/Variations*
Rossini, arr. Darnborough *Scenes from Cenerentola*
Peter Carr *Short Sonata No. 2*
Maurice Ravel *Jeux D'Eau*
Malcolm Dedman *Sonata No. 2 'In Search'*

Jonathan Darnborough (pno)

March 27

Alan Bullard *Dances for wind quintet; Three Bird
    Songs; Three Improvisations; Variations on an
    English Folk Song*
Timothy Torry *Two Nocturnes; Poem for Epiphany*
György Ligeti *Six Bagatelles*
Alan Parsons *Little Concerto for piano and wind
    quintet*

Balkerne Ensemble Wind Quintet, Alan Bullard,
Trevor Cordwell, Josephine Humbles (pnos),
Timothy Torry (bar)

April 1

Stravinsky, arr. Nankivell *Sonata for 2 pianos
    (2 movts)*
Rick Bolton *Pounding*
Dean Brodrick *Hoket*
Andrew Okrzeja *Canto 12*
Adrian Lee *My Man Mycool*
Hugh Nankivell *Trumpet Concerto (extract)*
Ellington, arr. Brodrick *Songs*
Anon *Sumer is icumen in* and *Estampie*

Was It A Car Or Cat I Saw? Ensemble

April 8

Benjamin Britten *Suite Op. 6 (Three Pieces)*
Krzysztof Penderecki *Three Miniatures*
Roger Steptoe *Study for solo violin*
Paul Patterson *Luslawice Variations*
Roy Teed *Elegy (In Memoriam Ralph Holmes);
    Tarantella* ☆☆☆
Benjamin Dale *Sonata*

Peter Sheppard (vln), Rupert Burleigh (pno)

April 10

Leon King; *Viola Duo* ☆☆☆
David Charles Martin *Lovers, for two violas* ☆☆☆*;
    Kisses for Mim; I am the Wind; Another Man's
    Word; Jack's Visit; Jugglin' Jack; Promotion 11*

Bridget Carey, Leon King (vlas), Penelope Mackay
(sop), David Charles Martin (pno), Gareth Roberts
(tenor)

April 14

John White *Gothic Chimes; Gothic Waltz; Piano
    Duets Nos. 1, 6, and 9 (1st set); Journey to the
    North Pole (film interlude); Duettino for flute
    and piano; Piano Sonatas Nos. 52, 55, and 96;
    Photocopying Machine; Air Today Gone
    Tomorrow; Yet Another Exercise; Heroic,
    Schlock, Waltz (Nordic Reverie Trio); Viking*

Birdbath; Waltz; Doggerel; 1st Sonatina for 2 tubas (March); Air Zaire's Heir's Heir's Ayre; Nocturnal Embarkation for Cyprus; Relaxation from the good works; Woman's Theme (Death of a Salesman); Grieg Takeaway; Loose Counterpoint with a strict lady; Mode 2 Machine; Toccata

Tributes to John White by Francis Shaw, John Tilbury, Howard Skempton, Adrian Jack, Keith Rowe and Eddie Prevost, Garry Judd, Ted Szanto, Hugh Shrapnel, Rick Morecambe, Ian Lake, Michael Nyman, Brian Dennis, Tony Godwin, John Lewis, Bryn Harris, Roddy Skeaping, Chris Hobbs, Warren Mitchell, Bob Briggs, Andrew Thomson, Osborne Peasgood, Pat Garrett, and Gavin Bryars

Fiftieth birthday celebration for John White devised by Ben Mason

April 15
Michael Tippett *Piano Sonata No. 4*
Ronald Stevenson *Passacaglia on DSCH*

Raymond Clarke (pno)

April 17
Harry Gilonis/John James *Lucretia Borgia*

Harry Gilonis (perc, toys), John James (tbn), Richard Barrett (guitar), David Preece (bn), Dafydd Thorne (live electronics)

April 28
Howard Haigh *Quidditty (two performances); What do you expect; The Secret Dreams of a Heronesque Affair; The Mummers Dance*
Ian Willcock *African Hours*

Collective Title; Fiona Baines (sop and perc), Howard Haigh (guitar and perc), Phil Halliwell and Ian Willcock (perc), Polly Hewett (vc), Clare Padley (fl)

April 30
Allan Moore *Uisgeachan; Notturno Raggiante*
Ian Morgan-Williams *Lyric Shadow*
Roberto Gerhard *Capriccio*
Aaron Copland *Duo*

Marion Ackrill (fl), Allan Moore (pno)

May 6
Hans Werner Henze *Sonatina* ☆
Stuart Bruce *Sonata* ☆
Denis Aplvor *Study for trombone* ☆☆☆
Martin Harvey *Processional (revised version)* ☆☆☆
George Nicholson *Slide Show*
Stephen Montague *Paramell I*
Reginald Smith Brindle *Tubal Cain's legacy*
Peter Maxwell Davies *Sonatina* ☆☆☆
Sohrab Uduman *Thrusts* ☆☆☆

Martin Harvey (tbn), Andrew Okrzeja (pno)

May 8
Dominic Muldowney *. . In a Hall of Mirrors . .*
Arnold Bax *Clarinet Sonata*
Giacinto Scelsi *Tre Pezzi* ☆☆
Francis Poulenc *Clarinet Sonata*

David Heath *Coltrane* ☆☆☆
Peter Seabourne *Roundelay (revised version)* ☆☆☆

Stephen Cottrell (sax), Jessica Drake (pno), Andrew Sparling (cls), Nicola Bibby (pno)

May 12
David Aldridge *Die Welt Des Schweigens*
Christopher Best *Piano Sonata – Reconciliations*
Philip Cashian *Nocturne*
Peter Graham *Moments for piano*

Michael Finnissy (pno)

May 13
York Bowen *Clarinet Sonata*
Janetta Gould *September for solo basset horn* ☆
Jean-Luc Darbellay *Espaces for solo basset horn* ☆☆
John Carmichael *Fetes Champêtres; Dance Suite*
Francis Poulenc *Clarinet Sonata*
Malcolm Macdonald *Cuban Rondo*

Marc Naylor (cl and basset horn), John Carmichael (pno)

May 15
Richard Dinnadge *Movement for string quartet*
Christopher Hobbs *Seventeen One Minute Pieces*
Michael Parsons *Highland Variations*
Benjamin Britten *String Quartet No. 3*

Goldsmiths' String Quartet

May 20
Pawlu Grech *Due movimenti; Ideograms – Book I; Ideograms – Book II; Quaderno I; Quaderno II; Continuous Contrasts*

Richard Deering (pno)

May 22
Ian Gardiner *21st century foxtrot; Satie's 'Trois Avant-Dernières Pensées'*
Andrew Thomson *A Slight List; White Epiphany*
Gavin Bryars *Ponukelian Melody; The Cross-Channel Ferry*

George W. Welch Ensemble

May 27
Frederick Delius *Three Preludes*
Toru Takemitsu *For Away; Piano Distance*
George Nicholson *Cascate*
Hugh Wood *Three Piano Pieces*
Per Nørgaard *Achilles and the Tortoise* ☆

John Byron (pno)

May 29
Malcolm Singer *For young ears only; Sonata for piano*
Manos Hadjidakis *For a little white seashell*
Erik Satie *Gnossienne No. 1; Le Piccadilly, Marche; Sur un casque; No. 3 de Podophthalma*

Christodolous Georgiades (pno)

June 3
Percy Grainger *Lord Maxwell's Goodnight; The power of love; David of the White Rock*

Benjamin Britten *Tit for Tat*
Peter Warlock *Candlelight*
David Dawson *Three Epitaphs* ☆☆☆
Richard Barrett *Principia*
Charles Ives *Religion; Feldeinsamkeit; Karen; The greatest man; The sideshow; In the alley*

Austin Allen (bar) Michael Finnissy (pno)

June 5
Mervyn Horder *Three Songs by Shakespeare; Five Songs by Robert Herrick; A Shropshire Lad; Heel and Toe, Rhythmic Dances; Four Songs by W. H. Auden; Four Songs by Charles Causley*
Geoffrey Wright *Songs for Senior Citizens*

Peter Allanson (bar), Stephen Betteridge (pno), Stephen Harris and Mervyn Horder (pno duet)

June 9
Bryan Kelly *Three Bagatelles*
David Dubery *Sonatine (after a poem by Verlaine)* ☆

Jonathan Tobutt (ob), David Leigh Dubery (pno)

June 16
John Michael Clarke *String quartet*
Richard Dinnadge *Movement for string quartet*
Michael Rosas-Cobian *Spells*

Fairfield String Quartet

June 17
György Ligeti *Six Bagatelles*
Aubert Lemeland *Quintette No. III* ☆☆
David Lancaster *Variations* ☆☆☆
Paul Patterson *Comedy for five winds*

Epsilon Wind Quintet

June 19
Mervyn Burtch *Sonatina No. 2*
Bernard Barrell *Five Piano Pieces for one hand*
Bernard Stevens *Ballad Op. 17*
Alan Bullard *Three Improvisations*
John McLeod *Piano Sonata No. 1*
Graham Whettam *Night Music*
Harry Samuels *Bagatelle*
David Nevens *Twelve Variations on a Polish Dance Melody*

Wanda Koseda (pno)

June 23
Franz Schubert *Andantino Varié in B minor D823; Rondo in A major D951*
Nicholas Carleton *Praeludium, A Verse*
Michael Blake *Impromptu* ☆☆☆
Claude le jeune, arr. Grainger *La Bel' Aronde*
Percy Grainger *Let's Dance Gay in Green Meadow; Harvest Hymn*
George Gershwin/Grainger *Embraceable You*
Richard Rodney Bennett *Capriccio*
Constant Lambert *Trois Pièces Nègres*
Billy Mayerl *Ace of Spades*

Michael Blake and Roy Stratford (pno duet)

July 1
John Ireland *Fantasy Sonata*
Richard Stoker *Partita*
John McCabe *Three Pieces*
Martin Ellerby *Sonata in Blue*

Linda Merrick (cl), Andrew Wilkinson (pno)

July 3
Robin Walker *age/a gita*
Javier Alvarez *Lluvia de Toritos*
Michael Parkin *Elegy*
Paul Archbold *Proteus*
Robert Keeley *Pastorale per la notte di natale* ☆☆☆
Philip Feeney *Watercolour*

Mandala, David Harvey (guitar), Nancy Ruffer (fl), Rupert Bawden (vla)

July 7
Pierre Boulez *Dérive*
Olivier Messiaen *Le Merle Noir*
Derek Foster *Intermediary*
Harrison Birtwistle *Verses for clarinet and piano*
Stefan Wolpe *Piece in two parts for six players*

Morley Musica Viva, directed by Michael Graubart

July 10
Frederick Delius *Violin Sonata No. 3*
Peter Warlock *Capriol Suite (arr. Szigeti)*
Edward Grieg *Sonata in C minor*
Antonin Dvořák *Four Romantic Pieces*

Roger Garland (vln), Angela Brownridge (pno)

July 17
York Bowen *Viola Sonata No. 1*
Robert Keeley *Sonata* ☆☆☆
Arthur Bliss *Sonata*
Leon King (vla), Robert Keeley (pno)

July 22
Anthony Green *Four Movements; Mosaic* ☆☆☆
Janet Graham *A Little Duet for James and Mary* ☆
Anthony Gilbert *Piano Sonata No. 2*
Derek Foster *Two Chrysalids* ☆☆☆
Frank Bayford *Sonata No. 2*
Richard Rodney Bennett *Capriccio*

Derek Foster and Anthony Green (pno duet)

July 24
Michael Jacques *Elegy and Burlesque*
Anthony Hedges *Sonata*
Catherine Kiernan *Duo for cello and piano*
Thomas Wilson *Fantasia for solo cello*
Antoinette Kirkwood *Sonata*

Alfia Nakipbekova (vc), Ray Holder (pno)

July 28
Frank Merrick *Tagomezo; La Cisterno; Somero Nokto; Oktobro; Ocean Lullaby*
Margaret Lyell *Verses to Music; Nightshade; 'Twas now the earliest morning*

Ronald Stevenson *Nocturne 'Hommage to John Field'; Traighean; Herbst; The Song of the Nightingale; The Lea*
Jules Massenet *Valse treslente; Two Impromptus; Dormons parmi les lis; Plus vite; Soir de rêve; Rêverie sentimentale; Il pleuvait; Berceuse; Au tres aime; Rondel de la belle au bois*

Stella Wright (mezzo-sop), Margaret Lyell (pno)
Ronald Stevenson (pno)

July 29
E. J. Moeran *Stalham River*
Herbert Howells *Gadabout*
Richard Rodney Bennett *Scena 1*
Timothy Seddon *Theme and Seven Variations*
Michael Zev Gordon *Three Pieces* ☆
Arthur Bliss *Triptych*
Lord Berners *Trois Petites Marches Funèbres*

Roger Steptoe (pno)

July 31
Roberto Gerhard *Three Impromptus*
Zsolt Durko *Son et lumière* ☆☆
Justin Connolly *Ennead; Night Thoughts*
György Kurtag *Splitter*
Simon Holt *Piano Piece*
Béla Bartók *Suite 'Out of Doors'*

Stephen Gutman (pno)

August 5
Havergal Brian *Prelude and Fugue in C minor; Prelude and Fugue in D minor/major; Double Fugue in E flat*
Peter Dickinson *Paraphrase II*
Carl Nielsen *Piano Piece in C; Three Pieces; Chaconne*
Niels Viggo Bentzon *Passacaglia*
Allan Pettersson *Lamento*

Raymond Clarke (pno)

STEPHEN PLAISTOW
Chief Producer, Contemporary Music, BBC Radio 3

BBC Radio 3 Music in Our Time

This series of weekly programmes on Radio 3 is broadcast on Thursday evenings at ten o'clock, and runs throughout the year with a break of two months in the summer during the season of Henry Wood Promenade Concerts. The aim is to include a maximum of variety of vital new work and a minimum of dogma, with some emphasis on what is radical and exploratory.

But the series is not only a forum for the very new. It fulfils the function of offering 'another chance to hear' and of promoting revivals of works which may have been admired when first performed and which now stand in need of fresh assessment and illumination by new programme contexts. It acknowledges that there is new music of good quality which was written longer ago than yesterday and which deserves to be performed and listened to more than once. Listeners to the programmes can expect to find established international masters who have achieved recognition in the last 25 years or so side by side with younger generations of composers who are acquiring their own mastery. There is room for surveys of many different territories, large and small, and for editions or mini-retrospectives devoted to individuals. The programmes make a point of reflecting what is going on outside Great Britain and try to bring to the radio listener here worthwhile new music wherever it may be found.

The programmes stand or fall by their success as radio broadcasts. Some half a dozen producers up and down the land contribute to the series regularly, but it is by no means a ghetto and those who make the programmes are not assuming to be reaching an audience of only music students and 'trade'. The styles of presentation are varied, and the spoken word in each programme aims to be informative, concise, appropriate, and written and delivered in such a way as to make the listener want to stay and listen to the music. There is plenty of room for expressions of opinion – without which the music would not have been chosen – and a recognition that the most stimulating and authoritative broadcasting about new music often comes from composers themselves, though not necessarily when talking about their own music.

There are no quotas for new music on Radio 3, or for any other commodity. Programmes are accepted by the network controller through an editorial process of debate at regular meetings which all producers are free to attend. It is the producers who are paid to have ideas and to turn them into programmes. In supplying programmes, the concern of the Radio 3 Music Department is to find the most pragmatic way of achieving the right balance between three kinds of operation: the promotion of the BBC's own programmes, the reflection of events promoted by others, and the occasional co-operation with other promoters – at the Huddersfield and Almeida Festivals, for example – in the interest of projects which can only be developed jointly and which require Radio 3's involvement from the beginning. A particular concern in recent years has been to give Radio 3's own activities a high profile by packaging contemporary music attractively and by identifying projects which only the resources of a large broadcasting organization could make possible. This is proving to be successful. There is no doubt that among the many 'minorities' which make up the Radio 3 audience the one for new music is growing.

The *Music in Our Time* programmes list covers the 1985–6 season, to which the special series of 'IRCAM in London' and 'Boulez at 60' (also listed) were a complement. This of course represents only part of Radio 3's output of new music during that period. The picture was enhanced by the BBC's public concerts, arguably the most important part of it and certainly the most visible – and the only part the newspapers usually notice – and completed by 'mixed' programmes (i.e., those in which contemporary music shared the bill with other works) too numerous to itemize.

September 19
Steve Reich *Music for eighteen musicians*

Steve Reich and musicians
Gramophone record

September 26
Peter Nelson *Zerissen . . .!*†
Gilles Tremblay *Envoi, for orchestra with piano solo*†

Timothy Blackmore (pno), Contemporary Chamber Orchestra, Odaline de la Martinez (director)
BBC studio recording

October 3
Claude Vivier *Lonely child*†
Steve Martland *Lotta continua*†

Pauline Vaillancourt (sop), Contemporary Chamber Orchestra, Odaline de la Martinez (director)
BBC studio recording

October 10
Hans Abrahamsen *Nacht und Trompeten*†
Per Nørgaard *Symphony No. 3*

Danish Radio SO, directors Sixten Ehrling (Abrahamsen), Tamàs Vetö (Nørgaard)
Danish Radio recording

October 17
Poul Ruders *Manhattan Abstraction*†
Ib Nørholm *Symphony No. 7 (Ecliptic instincts)*†

Danish Radio SO, director Michael Schønwandt (Ruders)
Danish Radio recording
Royal Danish Orchestra, director Leif Segerstram (Nørholm)
Gramophone record

October 24
John Casken *To fields we do not know* ☆☆☆
John Casken *Orion over Farne*

BBC Singers, conductor John Poole (To fields)
SNO, Matthias Bamert (director)
BBC recordings

October 31
Iannis Xenakis *Atrées*
Tristan Murail *Ethers*†
Gérard Grisey *Périodes*†
Jean-Pierre Guézec *Architectures colorées*

Ingrid Culliford (fl) (Murail), Lontano, Odaline de la Martinez (director)
BBC recording

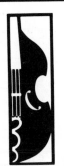

November 7
Jean-Pierre Guézec *Onze pour cinq*†
Maurice Ohana *Signes*☆☆
James Dillon *East 11th St NY 10003*†

Ingrid Culliford (fl), Paul Roberts (pno), Monique Rollin (zithers) (Ohana), Lontano, Odaline de la Martinez (director)
BBC recording

November 14
Enrique Pinilla *5 pieces for percussion*†
Naresh Sohal *Surya*
Poul Ruders *Régime for 3 percussionists* ☆☆
Michael Finnissy *Haiyim* ☆☆☆
Jennifer Fowler *Echoes from an antique land* ☆☆☆
Michael Finnissy *Ngano*

Sebastian Bell (fl), James Holland, David Johnson, David Hockings (perc), Alexander Baillie, Melissa Phelps (vcs), Judith Bingham (mezzo-sop), Neil Mackenzie (tenor), London Percussion Ensemble, Oliver Knussen (director), BBC Singers, Simon Joly (director)
BBC studio recordings

November 21
Chris Dench *Enoncé* ☆☆
Rolf Gehlhaar *Sub rosa*†; *Particles*†
Luigi Nono *Con Luigi Dallapiccola* ☆☆

Catherine Bott (sop), Michael Finnissy (pno), Alan Brett (vc), Music Projects/London, Richard Bernas (director)
BBC studio recording

November 28
Niccolo Castiglioni *Tropi*
Franco Donatoni *Lumen*
Aldo Clementi *Berceuse* ☆☆
Sylvano Bussotti *Tramonto* ☆☆
Salvatore Sciarrino *Centauro marino* ☆☆

Divertimento Ensemble, Milan, Sandro Gorli (director)
BBC recording (from the 1985 Huddersfield Festival)

December 5
Luciano Berio *Coro*

BBC Singers, BBC SO, Luciano Berio (director)
BBC studio recording

December 12
Luciano Berio *Requies* ☆☆; *Corale; Folk Songs; Voci*

Carlo Chiarappa (vln), Aldo Bennici (vla), London Sinfonietta Voices, London Sinfonietta, Luciano Berio (director)
BBC recording (from Queen Elizabeth Hall concert the same evening)

December 19
Jonathan Harvey *Concelebration*
Bernard Rands *Canti del sole* (chamber version) †
John Hopkins *White Winter, Black Spring* ☆☆☆

Martyn Hill (tenor), Henry Herford (bar), Lontano, Odaline de la Martinez (director)
BBC recording (from the 1985 Huddersfield Festival)

December 26
Margaret Sambell *Metal harmonics*
David Jaffe *Silicon Valley Breakdown*†
Charles Amirkhanian *Church Car II*†
Stephen Montague *Overture to I, Giselle*†
Charles Dodge *Any resemblance is purely coincidental*†
David Koblitz *How to Pachanga*†

Recent electro-acoustic pieces – composers' tapes and BBC studio recording

1986

January 9
György Kurtàg *Messages of the late Miss R. V. Troussova*
Harrison Birtwistle . . . *agm* . . .

Adrienne Csengery (sop), Marta Fabian (cimbalom), Ensemble Intercontemporain, director Pierre Boulez (Kurtàg) gramophone record
John Alldis Choir, Ensemble Intercontemporain, director Pierre Boulez
(Birtwistle) gramophone record

January 16
Colin Griffith *First book of spells* ☆☆☆
James Clarke *Kväll*†
Stephen Kings *Phantasy V* ☆☆☆
Rhian Samuel *Shadow Dance* ☆☆☆
Andrew Vores *Humming Harvest Gone snow motor* ☆☆☆

Capricorn, Lionel Friend (director)
BBC recording (of SPNM concert, St John's, Smith Square)

January 23
David Mott *A little small-talk*†
Ingram Marshall *Fog Tropes*†
Lars Sandberg *Touch*†
Poul Ruders *Four dances in one movement*†

David Mott (bar sax) (Mott)
Mats Persson and Kristine Scholz (two pnos) (Sandberg)
Danish Radio SO, director Oliver Knussen (Ruders)
Tapes from overseas radio organizations

January 30
Roger Reynolds *Transfigured Wind III*†
Paul Lansky *As if*†
Judith Weir *The Consolations of Scholarship*†

Ingrid Culliford (fl) (Reynolds),
Linda Hirst (mezzo-sop) (Weir),
Javier Alvarez (sound projection) (Lansky),
Lontano, Odaline de la Martinez (director)
BBC recording

February 6
Richard Rodney Bennett *Commedia II*

Erika Fox *Quasi una cadenza*†
Judith Weir *Several Concertos*†

Lontano, Odaline de la Martinez (director)
BBC recording

February 13
Heinz Holliger *Scardanelli Cycle (part 1)*†

Aurèle Nicolet (fl), Schola Cantorum, Stuttgart
South-West German Radio Symphony Orchestra,
Heinz Holliger (director)
South-West German Radio recording (from the
1985 Donaueschingen Festival)

February 20
Poul Ruders *Corpus cum Figuris*†
Unsuk Chin *Spektra*†
Ton Bruynel *Denk mal das Denkmal*†
Louis Andriessen *Velocity*†

Netherlands Radio Chamber Orchestra, conductor
Ernest Bour (Ruders), Taco Kooistra, Viola de
Hoog, Edvard van Regteren Altena (vcs) (Chin),
Lieuwe Visser (bar) (Bruynel), Netherlands Radio
SO, director Lucas Vis (Andriessen)
Netherlands Radio recordings (from the 1985
ISCM World Music Days)

February 27
James Clarke *Forsvinna*†
Klaus Huber *. . . Nudo que ansi juntais . . .*
Helmut Lachenmann *Mouvement – vor der
    Erstarrung*†
Enrique Raxach *Vortice*†
Michael Torke *Vanada*†

Harry Sparnaay (b cl), Netherlands Radio Chamber
Orchestra, director Ernest Bour (Clarke),
Netherlands Radio Choir, director Robin Gritton
(Huber), Ensemble Modern, director Lothar
Zagrosek (Lachenmann), The Bass Clarinet
Collective (Raxach), ASKO Ensemble, director
Lucas Vis (Torke)
Netherlands Radio recordings (from the 1985
ISCM World Music Days)

March 6
Michael Rosenzweig *Symphony in one movement*†
Steve Martland *Babi Yar*†

RLPO, Nicholas Cleobury (director)
BBC recording (of SPNM event in the Barbican
Hall, London)

March 13
Eric Stokes *Wondrous World*†
John Buller *Kommos*†
Arne Nordheim *Aurora*†

Electric Phoenix
BBC studio recording

March 20
John Marlow Rhys *Two Portraits* ☆☆☆
Jonathan Harvey *Song Offerings* ☆☆☆
Elliott Schwartz *Spirals* ☆☆☆

Rosemary Hardy (sop) (Harvey), Elliott Schwartz
(pno) (Schwartz), Spectrum, Guy Protheroe
(director)
BBC recording (from Queen Elizabeth Hall concert)

March 27
Harrison Birtwistle *Carmen arcadiae mechanicae
    perpetuum; Words overheard*†*; Earth dances*

Penelope Walmsley Clarke (sop), SCO, Harrison
Birtwistle (director), BBC SO, director Peter Eötvös
(Earth dances)
BBC studio recordings

April 3
Lukas Foss *Salomon Rossi Suite*†*; Night Music for
    John Lennon*†*; Baroque Variations*

Equale Brass, BBC Welsh SO, Lukas Foss
(director)
BBC studio recording

April 10
Elisabeth Lutyens *Six*†
Theo Lovendie *Music for contrabass and piano*†
Will Eisma *Gesang XXIII*†
Lyell Cresswell *Organic Music*†
Karlheinz Stockhausen *Set sail for the sun*
Roger Dean *Heteronomy 3*†
A group improvisation

Lysis, directors John Wallace and Roger Dean
BBC studio recording

April 17
Michael Finnissy *Câtana*†
Gwyn Pritchard *Lollay, lollay*†
Alain Bancquart *Ma manière d'oiseau*†

Uroboros, directors Gwyn Pritchard (Pritchard and Bancquart) and Michael Finnissy (Finnissy)
BBC recording

April 24
Alfred Schnittke *Piano Quintet*
David Blake *Clarinet Quintet*
György Ligeti *Horn Trio*

Capricorn
BBC recording

May 1
György Ligeti *Double concerto for flute and oboe; Ramifications; Melodien*

Douglas Townshend (fl), David Cowley (pno), BBC Welsh SO, Odaline de la Martinez (director)
BBC studio recording

May 8
György Ligeti *San Francisco Polyphony*
York Höller *Piano Concerto*
David Matthews *In the dark time*

Peter Donohoe (pno), BBC SO, directors Elgar Howarth (Ligeti and Höller) and Mark Elder (Matthews)
BBC studio recording

May 15
Marek Kopelent *String Quartet No. 5; Concertino for cor anglais and ensemble; Agnus Dei for soprano and ensemble*

Suk Quartet, Jiri Hebda (CA), Sigone von Osten (sop), Prague Chamber Ensemble, Bohumil Kulinsky (director)
West German Radio recording

June 12
Barry Anderson *Sound the tucket sonance and the note to mount, for tenor trombone and tape*†*; Proscenium*†
Harrison Birtwistle *Chronometer*

James Fulkerson (tbn), Simon Limbrick (perc), West Square Electronic Music Ensemble, director Barry Anderson
BBC studio recordings

June 19
Harrison Birtwistle *Monody for Corpus Christi*
Erika Fox *Paths where the mourners tread*†
George Mowat-Brown *Elogium*†

Jane Manning (sop), Lontano, director Odaline de la Martinez (Birtwistle and Fox) and George Mowat-Brown (Mowat-Brown)
BBC studio recording

June 26
Barbara Kolb *Three Place Settings*†
Pozzi Escot *Visone*†

Barbara Kolb *Homage to Keith Jarrett and Gary Burton*
Gloria Coates *Five Pieces for four wind players*†
Barbara Kolb *Chromatic Fantasy*†

Elaine Barry (sop), Gary Raymond (narrator), Lontano, Odaline de la Martinez (director)
BBC studio recording

July 3
Peter Maxwell Davies *Runes from a holy island*
Bayan Northcott *Six Japanese Lyrics* ☆☆☆
Ross Edwards *Laikaan*†
Bayan Northcott *Sextet*†

Sarah Leonard (sop), The Fires of London, directors Peter Maxwell Davies (Maxwell Davies) and Nicholas Cleobury (Northcott and Edwards)
Gramophone record and BBC studio recording

July 10
Stefan Wolpe *Second Piece for violin alone; Passacaglia for piano; Sim Shalom, Lilacs, Epitaph (Songs from the Hebrew); Form for piano; Chamber Piece No. 1 for 14 players*

Marilyn Dubow (vln), Garrick Ohlsson (pno) (Passacaglia), Russell Sherman (pno) (Form), Emilie Berendson (mezzo-sop), David Bloch (pno), Contemporary Chamber Ensemble, Arthur Weisberg (director)
Gramophone records and BBC studio recordings

July 17
Stefan Wolpe *Tango; Suite im Hexachord for oboe and clarinet; Enactments for three pianos*†

Yvar Mikhashoff (pno), Darrel Randall (ob) and Floyd Williams (cl), Cheryl Seltzer, Anne Chamberlain and Joel Sachs (pnos)
Gramophone records and BBC studio recording

IRCAM in London

Three programmes of electro-acoustic music from the first 10 years of the Institut de Recherche et Co-ordination Acoustique/Musique: presented by Radio 3 at St John's, Smith Square, London in October 1985.

May 18
Tristan Murail *Désintégrations*
Nigel Osborne *Alba*
York Höller *Arcus*

Linda Hirst (mezzo-sop), London Sinfonietta, Peter Eötvös (director)

May 22
Jean-Baptiste Barrière *Chréode I*
John Chowning *Stria*
Tod Machover *Soft morning, city!*
Jonathan Harvey *Mortuos plango, vivos voco*

Jane Manning (sop) and Barry Guy (cb) (Machover)

May 27

Gilbert Amy *La variation ajoutée*
Philippe Manoury *Zeitlauf*

BBC Singers, London Sinfonietta, Peter Eötvös
(director)

Hommage A Pierre Boulez

Three programmes of his music presented as a 60th
birthday tribute last year at Baden-Baden by the
South-West German Radio.

May 21

Pierre Boulez *Le marteau sans maître; Livre pour
cordes*

Elizabeth Laurence (mezzo-sop), Ensemble
Intercontemporarain, director Pierre Boulez (Le
marteau) New Philharmonia Orchestra, director
Pierre Boulez
(Gramophone record)

May 25

Pierre Boulez *Notations; Sonata No. 3; Structures,
Book II*

Pi-Hsein Chen (pno), Bernhard Wambach (pno)

May 29

Pierre Boulez *Répons*

Marta Fabian (cimbalom), Romi Ogawa-Helferich
(xylophone and glockenspiel), Andreas Boettger
(vibraphone), Yukiko Sugawara (pno and electric
org), Gunilde Cramer (pno), Ursula Holliger (hp),
South-West German Radio SO, Peter Eötvös
(director)

CHRISTOPHER FOX

Plural Darmstadt
The 1986 International Summer Course

Darmstadt must be Europe's most intensive new music festival: on each of the 15 days of the 1986 *Ferienkurse* there were lectures, seminars, classes, and listening sessions from nine in the morning until six in the evening when the concerts began, two and often three a night, finishing around midnight. It must be said immediately that some of the music heard was quite dreadful, so dreadful that one composer said to me that Darmstadt seemed to function as a Hoover, vacuuming up all the worst new music from Europe and America. On the other hand, it must also be said immediately that amongst the dross was some of the most stimulating and exciting new music to be heard anywhere.

In 1986, as in 1984, Friedrich Hommel structured the courses on a model of benign anarchy. A programme book was published, listing the main events of the fortnight, but (apart from the main evening concerts, which stayed much as advertised) these were often moved and, day by day, new events were added as they were proposed by the guest composers and fee-paying participants. Such an organizational model can produce frustrations, as I found when Morton Feldman, blissfully unaware of the passage of time, overran his allotted period by more than an hour and temporarily shunted both me and Chris Dench out of the schedule. But amazingly, by the end of the courses, most of the events proposed had actually happened – a considerable achievement for Hommel, and for Brian Ferneyhough, who was in charge of co-ordinating the lecture programme.

The intensive nature of the *Ferienkurse* means, inevitably, that it is a logistic impossibility to attend every session. This, coupled with the fact that I arrived 4 days late and also spent quite a lot of time in rehearsals, means that this review can make no claims to be comprehensive. This is not, however, entirely inappropriate to Friedrich Hommel's concept of the new Darmstadt, which he views as a mirror of the pluralism of today's new music. Furthermore, he believes that the 'private'

Darmstadt of informal conversation over food and drink is as important as the 'public' Darmstadt of the daily lecture programme, a further move away from the monolithic Darmstadt of the past and a further bar to the compilation of reviews which can claim to be comprehensive.

If the most realistic view of the new music world today is one which acknowledges the pluralist nature of that world, then Darmstadt is surely right to attempt also to be pluralistic in its policy for inviting musicians. Consequently, in 1986 there were appearances by composers as various as Michael Nyman, Trevor Wishart, Alvin Curran, Morton Feldman, Alain Bancquart, and Helmut Lachenmann. It is, of course, easy to suggest an even more diverse selection (one man's pluralism is another man's insularity) but conversations with a number of people seemed to confirm my feeling that the net might be cast wider still and ought especially to include a major Japanese composer. One notable omission was any composer with a direct connection with the old serial Darmstadt; nor was any of the music from that era performed. At one level, this is quite understandable – we live in a brave, new, uncertain world – but the time has perhaps arrived when a reassessment of work which, after all, constitutes a significant part of the recent history of music in Europe, would be fruitful for both composers and performers.

The sort of breadth of awareness which was evidently behind the assembly of the programme for 1986 seemed also to inform much of the best music that I heard. Nowhere was this more evident than in the music of Michael Finnissy, who was, with Brian Ferneyhough, the senior member of a large British contingent (amongst the others performed were James Dillon, Richard Emsley, James Erber, and Paul Robinson). There were performances of his String Quartet (1984) (the Arditti Quartet), *The Eureka Flag* (1983) (Nancy Ruffer), *English Country-Tunes* (1979) (Finnissy himself), *Duru-duru* (1981), and *Contretänze* (1985) (both by Exposé), of which the last two were new to me. Both these pieces share with the Quartet a fondness for formal outlines in which individual sections are very clearly differentiated from one another, not only by procedural changes but also, and more strikingly, by vivid changes in texture. If at times this sectionality works against a sense of any macro-structural process – I noted in myself a tendency to pay less attention to sections which did not particularly interest me, confident that soon enough something more attractive would come along – then Finnissy's sinuous melodies and his uninhibited invention of new instrumental combinations (the bass drum and castanet percussion writing at the start of *Duru-duru* is one memorable example of the latter, the viola melody somewhere in the middle of the Quartet an example of the former) are delightful compensations.

The Finnissy Quartet was one of the few pieces played by either of the string quartets in residence (the Kronos Quartet was the other one) that I would want to hear again. The depths of inanity were plumbed most thoroughly by Terry Riley's *Salome Dances for Peace* (1985–6) – an interminable, rambling piece of hokum 'inspired', the composer writes, 'by a vision of Kronos playing intricate passages on exotic scales and melodies together with precise and beautiful dancing offered in the spirit of peace and goodwill to all the creatures of the blue planet'. Perhaps with dance to distract attention from the banality of these 'intricate passages' – which were in reality no more exotic than the pastiche Dvořák of some facile but undisciplined student – the piece might just be tolerable; the concert version drove me out in just over half an hour.

Only in Wolfgang Rihm's Seventh Quartet (1986) did the Kronos find a work worthy of their beautifully blended sound and fine ensemble playing. Rihm's music always has a wilful spontaneity of organization, a sense that the music may go in whatever direction its composer's mood suggests, and the Seventh Quartet is a particularly playful and wayward construction. The whole work is triggered by the first violinist striking a woodblock, and woodblocks are used by all the players at some point in the piece, especially when the cello embarks on a wild solo that the other players attempt to disrupt with increasingly frenzied percussive activity. This cello cadenza has a curious counterpart at the work's close when the post-Bergian chromaticism of the rest of the piece gives way to an insistently repeated little tonal riff, again for cello, which seems to have no connection with anything else in the piece. For many people

this was just another irritant in an irritating work; I found it exhilarating – in this and Rihm's other quartets (the Ardittis played both *'Blaubuch'*, the Sixth Quartet (1984), and *Zwischenblick – Selbstthenker* (1984)) – to experience the results of an evidently manic creativity. At the same time, this is disturbing music – disturbing in that its composer's creativity seems happy to express nothing more than its own energetic abundance.

An altogether more considered approach was adopted by Carolyn Steinberg in her String Quartet No. 1 (1985), which the Ardittis premièred in their second concert. This is a beautifully crafted work, in an almost 'classical' post-serial idiom, whose material is subtly differentiated and as subtly developed. In the context of Darmstadt's four evenings of new music for string quartet it was almost unique in its restraint (for once, here was a composer who did not feel it imperative to run through the entire timbral gamut) and in its formal sophistication.

If Steinberg's quartet was based on the notion of the quartet medium as an essentially private one, then Michael Nyman's String Quartet (1985) was at the polar opposite, using amplification to emphasize its public nature. Curiously, this did not seem necessary, since the work's predominant gestural vocabulary – lots of virtuoso double-stopping in the upper regions – placed it quite clearly in the public domain. The main result of the amplification was that the extreme technical difficulty of the piece was made all too evident: both intonation and rhythmic ensemble were often erratic. In the Darmstadt atmosphere of 1982 (the year of my first visit) this piece would undoubtedly have caused a scandal with its regular rhythms and, worse still, its superficially banal tonal harmony; in 1986 it was well received (although it was conveniently placed at the end of the concert so that those unlikely to appreciate it could leave). I enjoyed Nyman's construction of an elaborate mosaic out of variants on John Bull and Schoenberg (although there is scope for a cut or two), yet I remained unconvinced that this material is best suited to the string quartet. But perhaps in the hands of players who had not just ploughed through ninety minutes of *ernstlichkeit* the work might sound less strenuous.

Darmstadt's most performed composer was Giacinto Scelsi, to whom a whole day was devoted. In the morning Martin Zenck lectured, drawing primarily on the piano music for his examples and demonstrating Scelsi's development from twelve-note composition to the use of pitch centres prevalent in the more recent music. In the afternoon Harry Halbreich played new recordings of some of the orchestral music; the evening concert concentrated on music from the late fifties onwards, mostly for one or two instruments but concluding with an ensemble piece, *Pranam I*, directed by Aldo Brizzi. Perhaps inevitably there is a sameness of gesture and structure in many of the solo pieces which makes such a sequence of them either tiresome or – for me, on this occasion – quite hypnotic. The trance was broken twice: eventually by the dignified passion of *Pranam*, but first by *For the Master* (1974), a duo for cello and piano which is striking in Scelsi's recent output for its avoidance of microtonal intervals and for its unambiguous harmonic organization. Where most of Scelsi's music since the *Quattro Pezzi* for orchestra (1956) relies on quarter-tone inflected lines shifting across one another, *For the Master* employs real two-part counterpoint (the piano writing is always in octaves) and does so with a boldness characteristic of its composer.

Pranam was encored, as were Robert HP Platz's *Flötenstücke* (1982–3) for solo alto flute (Pierre-Yves Artaud) and seven players, conducted by the composer. Like all Platz's recent music, the *Flötenstücke* deal with clearly articulated musical processes, but processes which are couched in the vocabulary of modernism and which have none of the predictability of much minimalist music. In the recently completed opera ... *Verkommenes Ufer* (1983–6), for example, there is a progression from the music for solo singers and chamber ensemble of the opening scene (premièred at Darmstadt in Ensemble Modern's opening concert) to, eventually, music for solo singers, chorus, orchestra, and tape, while the first of the *Flötenstücke* – which lasts for almost half of the work's ten minute duration – is dominated by the soloist, moving from long notes to ever shorter notes, at which point he is joined in rapid succession by bass flute, bass clarinet, and trumpet; then the process abruptly stops and the second movement begins.

The other pieces to capture my interest were also for ensemble. José Evangelista's *Clos de vie* (1983) I had heard on tape on Darmstadt in 1984 and memory suggests that the performance on that recording was more successful than that given live in 1986 by Ensemble Modern. The work is scored for five strings, harp, banjo, electric guitar, piano, harpsichord, and percussion, with much play being made of the timbral links between the plucked and keyboard instruments. The music is essentially monodic but Evangelista gives it a complex heterophonic orchestration, so that the cyclical melody on which it is based is constantly

diffused through rhythmic dislocations and through the glittering instrumental spectrum he has assembled. The piece closes with a quotation from *Lonely Child* by Claude Vivier, whom Evangelista's piece (especially its punning title) commemorates. Unfortunately, this was a rather monochromatic performance, due largely to inadequate amplification of the harpsichord. (The same was true of Richard Barrett's *Anatomy* (1985–6), premièred in the same concert, which the amplification rendered into a rather indigestible soup.)

Each Darmstadt asserts its own particular personality in the studio concerts which conclude the Ferienkurse and which provide the opportunity for the instrumental participants to perform the work of guest and participant composers. There was the usual quota of frenetic solo pieces, the most successful being Bernfried Pröve's violin piece *Firebird* (1986) and Bernardo Kuczer's *A-GENT'S ARGUUM* (1982) for viola (although for this listener the contest for best display vehicle had already been won by Roger Redgate's electric, slithering *Ausgangspunkte* (1981–2) for his oboist brother, Christopher Redgate). There were also some splendid performers in evidence, notably the violist Barbara Maurer in the Kuczer and the saxophonist, Pierre-Stéphane Meuge, in a number of pieces.

In 1984 the studio concerts had been reduced to little more than an exhaustive procession of such solo pieces, but in 1986 there were a refreshing number of ensemble pieces – a shift in emphasis achieved in part through better organization and in part through the energetic commitment of the members of the Arditti Quartet who appeared in piece after piece. The loveliest of the works played was probably Rod Sharman's *Erstarrung* (1984). Scored for nine instruments, this is a still, quiet sequence of chords which are attacked, revoiced, sustained, and then allowed to die away, the start of the next event depending on the decay time of the percussion and plucked instruments (harp, mandoline, and guitar) which form the nucleus of the ensemble.

The most arcane piece was, almost certainly, Klaus K. Hübler's *Feuerzauber* (1981) for three flutes, harp, and cello, all amplified. Hübler is a Ferneyhough pupil who has taken his teacher's ideas about parametric composition to extremes (Hübler's interpretation of these ideas is outlined in a recent article in Interface magazine): in this piece the amplification is needed to clarify precisely composed lip, breath, and finger activity, for example. A shortage of time for technical rehearsal obviously hindered this performance – the cello amplification was particularly unsatisfactory – and it may be that what emerged was not what the composer intended. However, I found the juxtaposition of the gravelly textures of cello and flutes and the pure-toned harp strings peculiarly entertaining.

After the pupil, the master. In 1984 five movements of Brian Ferneyhough's then incomplete *Etudes transcendentales* (1985) were performed in Darmstadt; in 1986 the remaining four of the now complete work were given. The *Etudes* (subtitled *Intermedio II*) form the fifth work in the *Carceri d'invenzione* cycle and are scored for mezzo-soprano, flute, oboe, amplified harpsichord, and cello with conductor (common to both Darmstadt performances were the singer Brenda Mitchell, flautist Pierre-Yves Artaud, cellist Alan Brett, and conductor Robert HP Platz). Clearly it is hard to get any sense of the whole in these circumstances, but what is clear is the resourcefulness of Ferneyhough's manipulation of his ensemble: the combination of voice and instruments is constantly changing, both between and within movements, with the whole ensemble only coming together in the fifth and ninth movements. If there is a disappointment in the work it is that in this, Ferneyhough's first work with solo voice, his treatment of the voice is so restrained. One consequence of this restraint is that while many points of contact – timbral, registral, and gestural – are established between the instruments, fewer are made between the rather sober vocal writing and the much wilder instrumental lines.

Again, the reception of the second instalment of the *Etudes* was interesting: in 1984 there was some booing; in 1986 there was only applause. If the tolerance shown in Darmstadt in 1986 was sometimes only superficial – there were still many instances of people refusing even to give a hearing to music they opposed – there was, none the less, a far less antagonistic atmosphere and a much greater openness. Long may the plural Darmstadt continue.

Chris Newman

Darmstadt

(meant to be) It is not that we are continually covering new ground, but rather that the old ground is constantly disappearing behind us our very eyes where we are, (facing backwards), Apart from the green of the ground holding (keeping it off with its greenness) up the low-hanging grey of the sky, meant to be thinking about Darmstadt, (the greenness radiating upwards is preventing the heavy low-hanging grey clouds with preventing them from touching the ground) the fact that I was meant to write my personal view of the Darmstadt Summer Course for New Music, writing about something other than about that is cheap, just chickening out, or is a genuine artistic approach or is both? (is both.).

The countryside is wild & outside & we are inside (the train) is like a town & yet the train is outside in the countryside & we are inside in the outside; Trains run (as if) by chance: It's not the train's fault that these houses were built. The main artistic concerns of a great piece of music have nothing to do with the superficial historical style of the piece for the composer at the time it is written, & yet it is this superficial historical style which has become the substance, the "concern", of the international English non-descript style composer of contemporary music; in other words, the work of this composer has no substance no heart is all emptiness. That which makes it all the more disturbing is this: that is, that the basic historical style which he/she has picked up, that is, Expressionism (Alban Berg), where style is a direct representation of highly personal emotion, this style has become institutionalised, the representation of somebody else's emotion has become

institutionalised, & masquerades now as a representation of the personal emotion of a non-descript composer, & thus all is totally false & never felt. This "non-descript" music consists of empty ready-made gestures (to fit the false emotions), which deprive those composers of expressing any real artistic concern(s) (even if they could), everything has been sacrificed for the sake of the gestures (which are empty); & these empty gestures, this music, can never be imbued with any substance by the non-descript composer because the n.-d. composer writes his/her work as if it were already written, from the point of view of the finished article, & so when he/she writes it, he/she writes all the music away that he/she started with (into emptiness), & we're—(they're)—left with nothing. (As the work itself is nothing, the sounds left over are totally redundant.) Thus it (the finished article) is unable to transcend what it started with, its own material, be more than its own material, transcend itself onto a higher spiritual level, & thus it cannot be a work of art. (The instrumentation of such pieces is a side-show of effects & "good ideas", which remain only effects & "good ideas" as such things only can, & have nothing to do with the work. It remains "instrumentation" which is separate from music, which adds to the redundant nature of the work.) This has become the way to write, what music is, has nothing to do with art, has become an easy & accepted way for so many to make a career, with each new generation feeding off the previous generation & thus becoming even more limited & stale than the previous; (the differences between the composers who write this kind of music are irrelevant).

International Music Information Centres

Australia
Room 405, 4th Floor, 3 Smail
  Street, Broadway 2007, Sydney
PO Box 49, Broadway 2007,
  Sydney
02 212 1611
Frank Maietta

Austria
Hanuschgasse 3, A-010 Wien
222 524299/523143
Dr Harald Görtz

Belgium
Rue d'Arlon 75–7, 1040 Bruxelles
02 2309430/2309437
Anna van Steenbergen

Canada
Chalmers House, 20 St Joseph
  Street, Toronto, Ontario,
  M4Y 1J9
416 961 6601
Simone Auger

Columbia
Calle 11, No. 5–51 Bogota 1
57 283 6903/282 8576
Maria Christina Sanchez

Czechoslovakia
Besedni 3, CS-11800 Praha 1
02 530546–8/539720
Dr Jan Ledec

Denmark
Vimmelskafret 48, DK-1161,
  Copenhagen K
01 112066
Knud Ketting

France
CDMC, 225 Avenue Charles de
  Gaulle, F-92521 Neuilly-sur-
  Seine, Paris
01 4747-5650
Marianne Lyon

Finland
Runebergsgatan 15 A 1,
  SF-00100 Helsinki 10
0409134/409707
Matti-Jussi Pollari

German Federal Republic
Nieder-Ramstadter Strasse 190,
  D-6100 Darmstadt
06151 132416/132417
Friedrich Hommel

Great Britain
10 Stratford Place, London W1N
  9AE
01 499 8567
Elizabeth Yeoman

Holland
Donemus, Paulus Potterstraat 14,
  1071 CZ Amsterdam
020 764436
Rogier Starreveld

Hungary
H-1364 Budapest, POB 47
V. Vorosmarty ter 1, Budapest
01 184-243
Hedvig Gergely

Iceland
PO Box 978, IS-121 Reykjavik
Freyjugötu 1, Reykjavik
01 21185
Karólína Eríksdóttir

Ireland
95 Lower Baggot Street, Dublin 2
01 762639/612105
Bernard Harris

Israel
PO Box 11253, IL-61112 Tel
  Aviv
6 Chen Boulevard, Tel Aviv
03 289514/284397
William Elias

Norway
Toftesgate 69, N-0552 Oslo 5
02 370909
Jostein Simble

Poland
Rynek Starego Miasta 27, PL-00-
  272 Warszawa
022 310607
Barbara Zwolska-Steszewska

Portugal
Fundacao Calouste Gulbenkian,
  Avenida de Berna 45, P-1093
  Lisboa
19 735131
*Maria Fernanda Cidrais
  Rodrigues*

Sweden
PO Box 273 27, S-102 54
  Stockholm
Sandhamnsgatan 79, Stockholm
08 783 8800
Roland Sandberg

Switzerland
Bellariastrasse 82, CH-8038,
  Zurich
01 482 6666
Hans Steinbeck

United States of America
250 West 54th Street, Room 300,
  New York NY 10019
212 247 3121
Nancy Clarke

Yugoslavia
PO Box 213, JU-11000 Beograd
Misarska 12–14, Beograd
11 344 254

Affiliated MICs

Scotland
7 Lilybank Gardens, Glasgow
  G12 8RZ
041 334 6393
John Purser

Wales
Music Department, University
  College, Corbett Road, Cardiff
  CF1 1XL
0222 44211
A. J. Heward Rhys

New Publications of British Music

The following, from several British publishers, list new works on sale or hire that have been published or contracted since August 1985.

Oxford University Press

HIRE

*denotes that a study score is available for sale

Chamber

Gerald Barry
  Sur Les Pointes
Michael Berkeley
  For the Savage Messiah
John Buller
  *Le Terrazze**
Edward Harper
  String Quartet
Anthony Powers
  *Chamber Concerto**
  *Quintet**
Robert Sherlaw Johnson
  *Projections**

Concerti

Gordon Crosse
  Array, concerto for trumpet and strings
William Mathias
  *Organ Concerto**

Orchestral

Michael Berkeley
  Daybreak and a Candle-end
John Buller
  *Proença**
  *The Theatre of Memory**
Martin Butler
  Cavalcade
  *The Flights of Col**
Gordon Crosse
  *Dreamsongs, Op. 43**
Edward Harper
  Fantasia V
Anthony Powers
  *Music for Strings**
  Vespers

Vocal

Michael Berkeley
  Songs of Awakening Love
John Buller
  Of Three Shakespeare Sonnets
  *The Mime of Mick, Nick, and the Maggies**
  *Two Night Pieces from Finnegans Wake**
Gordon Crosse
  A Wake Again
Edward Harper
  Caterwaul
  Hedda Gabler – opera, libretto on sale
Anthony Powers
  Venexiana

SALE

Richard Blackford
  Posthumous Leonatus – solo ob
John Buller
  Finnegans Floras – 14 voices, perc, pno
  Poor Jenny – fl and perc
  Scribenery – vc
Gordon Crosse
  Trio (Rhymes & Reasons) – cl, vc, pno
Alun Hoddinott
  Bagatelles – ob, hp
  Scena – string quartet
Anthony Powers
  Nocturnes, Book 2 – vc
  Sea/Air – cl

Chester Music

Geoffrey Burgon
  The Name of the Hare – unaccomp SATB chorus
  Orpheus – chamber opera
John Dankworth
  Suite for Emma – cl and pno
John Duarte
  Un petit jazz – fl or recorders and guitars
Dave Heath
  Out of the Cool – fl and pno

Witold Lutoslawski
  Partita – vln and pno
Robert Saxton
  Krystallen – fl and pno
Hugh Wood
  Paraphrase – cl and pno

The Chester Book of Carols
Seventeen carols, mostly for unaccompanied SATB, by leading contemporary composers, including Carol Barratt, Lennox Berkeley, Christopher Brown, Geoffrey Burgon, Brian Chapple, Witold Lutoslawski, Elizabeth Maconchy, Peter Maxwell Davies, Elizabeth Poston, Robert Saxton, John Tavener, and Hugh Wood.

Scores

Witold Lutoslawski
  Paganini Variations – pno and orch
Elizabeth Maconchy
  Music for Woodwind and Brass
Peter Maxwell Davies
  Birthday Music for John – chamber ensemble
  Into the Labyrinth – solo tenor and chamber orch
  The Lighthouse – chamber opera
  Quartet Movement – string quartet
  Sinfonia Concertante – chamber orch
  Sonatina for Violin and Cimbalom
  The Unbroken Circle – chamber ensemble

Boosey & Hawkes

Jonathan Lloyd
  Songs from the Other Shore cycle consisting of the following titles:
  It's all Sauce to me – vln and pno

Mill of Memories – cl and vc
Like Fallen Angels – fl, vla, and hp
Shorelines of Certainty – ensemble
Peter Maxwell Davies
First Ferry to Hoy
The Martyrdom of St Magnus
An Orkney Wedding, with Sunrise
Symphony No. 3
Andrzej Panufnik
Arbor Cosmica – for 12 solo strings
Concerto in Modo Antico

United Music Publishers

(WORKS PUBLISHED)

Simon Bainbridge
Music for Mel & Nora (1979) – ob and pno
Voicing (1982) – chamber ensemble

Richard Barrett
Coïgitum – chamber ensemble
Chris Dench
Caught Breath of Time – fl
Time – bass or bassett cl
Topologies – pno
Petr Eben
Desire of Ancient Things – unaccomp choir
Michael Finnissy
. . . Above Earth's Shadow – chamber ensemble
Banumbirr – chamber ensemble
Contretänze – chamber ensemble
English Country-Tunes – pno
Ngano – ST soloists, SATB choir, and 2 perc
Stephen Montague
Paramel VI – fl, cl, vc, and pno
Edwin Roxburgh
Quartet for Flute & Strings
Pierre Villette
Attende Domine – unaccomp SATB choir

United Music Publishers

(WORKS CONTRACTED)

Simon Bainbridge
Ceremony & Fanfare – brass and perc
Three Players (1985) – vc, bass cl, and pno

Richard Barrett
Anatomy – 11 instruments
Ne songe plus a fuir (1985–6) – vc
Chris Dench
Esperance – pno
Recueillement – 8 instrumentalists
Shunga – mezzo-sop and instrumental ensemble
Petr Eben
A Festive Voluntary on Good King Wenceslas – org
Landscapes of Patmos – org and 1 perc

Michael Finnissy
  String Trio
  Verdi Transcriptions – pno
Edwin Roxburgh
  Pianto – unaccomp SATB choir

Universal Edition, London

David Bedford
  Toccata in D minor – pno
Harrison Birtwistle
  Songs by Myself – sop and chamber ensemble
  Mask of Orpheus (libretto)
Earle Brown
  Centering – solo vln and chamber ensemble

Morton Feldman
  For Frank O'Hara – chamber ensemble
Michael Finnissy
  Mr Punch – voice and chamber ensemble
Simon Holt
  Mirrormaze – chamber ensemble
Vic Hoyland
  Serenade – chamber ensemble
Dominic Muldowney
  Saxophone Concerto
  Piano Trio
Nigel Osborne
  Mythologies – chamber ensemble
  Hell's Angels (libretto)
Paul Patterson
  Mean Time – brass quintet

Missa Brevis
Spiders
Luslawice Variations
Bernard Rands
  Cuaderno – string quartet
Peter Wiegold
  Sing Lullaby – sop and cb

For listings of composers, ensembles, and individual performers, consult either the *British Music Yearbook* (published by Rhinegold Publishing) or The British Music Information Centre, 10 Stratford Place, London W1N 9AE (tel. 01 499 8567); Centre Manager, Matthew Greenall, Information Services Manager, Tom Morgan.

 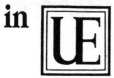

Listings of Selected Events

Festivals 1985–6

The following lists works by living British composers and first performances of works by foreign composers. Concert Series spread over several months are listed after individual festivals.

☆☆☆ First performance
  ☆☆ First British performance
    ☆ First London performance

Nettlefold Festival

Nettlefold Hall, 1 Norwood High Street, London SE27
Artistic Directors: Simon Deshorger and Lawrence Casserley

October 4
A performance by Nicholas Wilson (live and taped music with dancer)
Rolf Gehlhaar *Rondel* ☆☆
Arvo Pärt *Pari Intervallo* ☆☆
James Dillon *Parjanya-vata*

Music Projects/London, Richard Bernas (director)

October 5
Tristram Cary 60th-birthday concert
Priaulx Rainier *Cycle for Declamation*
Malcolm Hayes *Two Songs of Pablo Neruda* ☆
Simon Deshorger *Mugali* ☆☆☆
Karl Aage Rasmussen *Encore for Jane* ☆☆☆
Tristram Cary *Birth is Life is Power is Death is God is . . .; Narcissus; Nonet; Trellises* ☆☆; *I Am Here*

Jane Manning (sop), Simon Desorgher (fl), Tristram Cary (sound projection)

October 11
Douglas Doherty *Impact* ☆
Karlheinz Stockhausen; *Piano Piece XII* ☆
Justin Connolly *Ennead/Night Thoughts*
Simon Emmerson *Piano Piece IV* ☆
Alejandro Vinão *Go*
Ian Dearden *Kinesis*
Simon Emmerson *Time Past III*

Philip Mead (pno), Lawrence Casserley (sound projection)

October 12
Improvisation
Barry Guy (cb), Derek Bailey (guitar)

Pamela Smith *Fiddler's Dream*
Gordon Downie *Hi-Fi-Low-Fi*
George Robey *ID*
John Casken *Piper's Linn*

Richard Butler (Northumbrian smallpipes), Peter Manning (sound projection)

October 18
Invented Instruments Event
Hugh Davies and Hans-Karsten Raecke

October 19
Trevor Wishart *Vocalise 1*
Lawrence Casserley *Hydrangea*
Improvisation by Evan Parker (sax)

Random Access Ensemble and The Anglepoise Philharmonic

Huddersfield Festival

Huddersfield Polytechnic, Queensgate, Huddersfield HD1 3DH
Artistic Director; Richard Steinitz

November 19
Luciano Berio *Duetti* ☆☆
Michael Tippett *Concerto for Double String Orchestra*
Richard Steinitz *Canons for Violins* ☆☆☆

Chethams School of Music and local school children, Julian Clayton and Richard Steinitz (directors)

November 20
Geoffrey Poole *Ten*
Nicholas Sackman *Piano Sonata*

Peter Lawson (pno)

John Tavener *Trisagion* ☆☆☆
Philip Feeney *Thursday Night* ☆☆☆
James Ellis *Trying to fathom the paradox*
Richard Rodney Bennett *Commedia IV*
Tim Souster *Equalisation*

Equale Brass with Tim Souster (sound projection)

November 21
Jonathan Harvey *Transformations*
Judith Weir *Sketches from a Bagpiper's Album*
Jonathan Lloyd *True Refuge* ☆☆☆

Nicholas Cox (cl) and Vanessa Latarche (pno)

Elizabeth Maconchy *Quartetto Corto*

Fairfield Quartet

Bernard Rands *Cuardeno*
Franco Donatoni *The Heart's Eye* ☆☆
Michael Finnissy *String Quartet* ☆☆☆
Jonathan Harvey *String Quartet*

Arditti Quartet

November 22
John Marlow Rhys *Two Portraits*
Michael Finnissy *Banumbirr; Above Earth's Shadow* ☆☆☆
Jonathan Harvey *Song Offerings*

Spectrum with Rosemary Hardy (sop)
Guy Protheroe (director)
Jonathan Harvey *Concelebration*
Bernard Rands *Canti del Sole* ☆☆
John Hopkins *White Winter, Black Spring* ☆☆☆

Lontano with Martyn Hill (tenor) and Henry Herford (bar), Odaline de la Martinez (director)

Michael Finnissy *Nasiye*
Michael Tippett *The Blue Guitar*

Gerald Garcia (guitar)

November 23
Aldo Clementi *Berceuse* ☆☆
Sylvano Bussotti *Tramonto* ☆☆
Salvatore Sciarrino *Centauro Marino* ☆☆

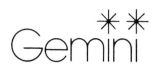

Divertimento Ensemble (Milan), Sandro Gorli (director)

Luciano Berio *Sequenza X for trumpet*

David Short (tpt)

November 24
Salvatore Sciarrino *Duetto* ☆☆☆
Ada Gentile *Come dal nulla* ☆☆
Brian Ferneyhough *Lemma-Icon-Epigram* ☆☆
Giacinto Scelsi *Kho-Lho* ☆☆☆
Brian Ferneyhough *Carceri d'Invenzione IIB* ☆☆☆
Giuseppe Soccio *Spirali* ☆☆
Luigi Nono *Inquietum* ☆☆
Aldo Clementi *Duetto con eco* ☆☆

Roberto Fabbriciani (fls), Ciro Scarponi (cls), Massimiliano Damerini (pno)

Dance and the Double Bass, an event by Chris Hill (dancer) and Sophie Preston (cb)

November 25
Salvatore Sciarrino *Comne vengono* ☆☆
Aldo Clementi *Fantasia su roBErto FABbriCiAni* ☆☆
Salvatore Sciarrino *Second Sonata for piano* ☆☆

Roberto Fabbriciani (fls) and Massimiliano Damerini (pno)

November 26
Bernard Rands *Déjà*
Giacinto Scelsi *Kya* ☆☆
Jonathan Harvey *Inner Light I*

Music Projects/London with Roger Heaton (cl), Richard Bernas (director)

November 27
Simon Emmerson *Time Past IV*
Jonathan Harvey *Nachtlied*
Michael Finnissy *Anninnia* ☆☆

Jane Manning (sop), David Mason (pno)

David Bedford *Sun Paints Rainbows on the Vast Waves*
Philip Wilby *Firestar*
Luciano Berio *Accordo* ☆☆

Local bands and twentieth-century ensembles directed by Adrian Baxter, David James, Major Peter Parks, Timothy Reynish, and Barrie Webb

Response
Music Box, Royal Festival Hall
London Sinfonietta, director Oliver Knussen
London Sinfonietta Voices, director Terry Edwards

November 29
Robin Holloway *Fantasy Pieces*

November 30
Oliver Knussen *Ophelia Dances; Autumnal; Three Little Fantasies for Wind Quintet; Masks*

December 1
Nigel Osborne *Choralis 1, 2, and 3*
Judith Weir *Serbian Cabaret*
Mark-Anthony Turnage *After Dark* ☆☆☆

Jonathan Lloyd *The Shorelines of Certainty* ☆☆
Poul Ruders *Wind-Drumming (revised version)* ☆☆☆

Park Lane Group – Young Artists and Twentieth-Century Music Series
Purcell Room

January 6
John McCabe *Variations*
Barry Guy *New work* ☆☆☆

Nicholas Unwin (pno), Rachel Brown (fl)

January 7
John McCabe *Three Pieces*
Michael Berkeley *Père du doux repos* ☆☆☆;
    Flighting ☆☆☆
Harrison Birtwistle *Verses for clarinet*
Peter Racine Fricker *Bagatelles* ☆☆

Jenny Miller (mezzo-sop), Nancy Cooley (pno),
Michael Whight (cl), James Lisney (pno)

January 8
Priaulx Rainier *Clarinet Suite*
Morris Pert *Luminos*
John McCabe *Requiem Sequence*
Elizabeth Maconchy *Three Songs*
Bernard Rands *Ballad III*

Duncan Prescott (cl), Scott Mitchell (pno), Tracey
Chadwell (sop), Pamela Lidiard (pno)

January 9
Peter Maxwell Davies *Trumpet Sonata*
Robert Harvey *Diversions* ☆☆
Javier Alvarez *Luz Caterpilar for piano and
    tape* ☆☆☆

Oren Marshall (tba), Vanessa Latarche (pno),
Andrew Crowley (tpt), David Mason (pno), Simon
Leben (pno)

January 10
Mark-Anthony Turnage; New work for saxophone
    and piano
Peter Maxwell Davies *The Kestrel Paced Round the
    Sun*
Duncan Fraser *Melodrama Compline*
John McCabe *Paraphrase on Mary Queen of Scots*
Kaikhosru Sorabji *Fantasie Espagnole*

Martin Robertson (sax), Anthony Gray (pno),
Victor Sangiorgio (pno), Katey Thomas (fl),
Graham Jackson (pno)

Almeida Theatre concerts
Almeida Street, London N1

January 26
Volker Heyn *Rozs* ☆☆
Christopher Fox *Etwas Lebhaft*
James Dillon *Zone (. . . de azul)* ☆☆☆
Hans Joachim Hespos *Esquisse Itineraire* ☆☆

Circle, Roger Heaton (director)

February 1
Mesias Maiguaschka *Monodias e Interludios* ☆☆
David Bedford *Visions of the Daughters of
    Albion* ☆☆☆
Michael Finnissy *Contretänze* ☆☆☆
Brian Bevelander *Fantasy Music* ☆☆

Singcircle and Circle, Gregory Rose (director)

February 2
Michael Finnissy *Ouraa* ☆☆☆
Giacinto Scelsi *Kya*
Chris Dench *Recueillement* ☆☆☆

Music Projects/London, Richard Bernas (director)

February 13
Dieter Schnebel *B dur* ☆☆
Erhard Grosskopf *Chamber Symphony* ☆☆;
    Katastrophenherz ☆☆

Music Projects/London, Richard Bernas (director)

City University Festival of Electro-acoustic Music
New Hall, Northampton Square, London EC1
Artistic Director; Simon Emmerson

February 25
Giacinto Scelsi *I presagi* ☆☆
Roger Smalley *Pulses; Echo III*

Music Projects/London with Graham Ashton (tpt),
Richard Bernas (director)

February 26
Simon Emmerson *Time Past IV*
Jonathan Harvey *Nachtlied*
Walter Fabeck *Circadian II*
Javier Alvarez *Luz Caterpilar*

Jane Manning (sop), David Mason (pno), Simon
Lebens (pno), The Fairer Sax (sax quartet)

February 27
Alejandro Viñao *Go*
Alan Belk *Tsuname*
Steve Stanton *Venetian Gondola Song*

Vocem, Frances Lynch (director)

Contemporary Chamber Orchestra
St John's, Smith Square

February 20
Bernard Benoliel *The Black Tower*
James Erber *Music for 25 Solo Strings* ☆☆☆

CCO, with Jane Manning (sop), Odaline de la
Martinez (director)

The Fires of London
Queen Elizabeth Hall

February 25
Peter Maxwell Davies *Seven in Nomine; Hymnos;
    Clarinet Sonata; Excuse Me, on old English
    ballads*

Philip Grange *Variations* ☆☆☆
Bayan Northcott *Sextet*

The Fires, Nicholas Cleobury (director)

York Spring Festival
York University
Artistic Director: Alan Hacker

March 7
Roger Marsh *Not a soul but ourselves*
Daryl Runswick *I sing the body electric*
Trevor Wishart *Vox 1 and 2*

Electric Phoenix

March 8
Stanley Hawkins *Clarinet Concerto* ☆☆☆
Arne Nordheim *Spur* ☆☆
Bernard Rands *Madrigali*

York University Chamber Orchestra with Jonty
Stockdale (cl), Gordon MacPherson (accordion),
and David Blake, John Godfrey, and Bernard
Rands (directors)

March 9
Michael Tippett *Quartet No. 2*
Peter Maxwell Davies *Little Quartet No. 1*
Robert Simpson *Quartet No. 10*

Coull String Quartet

March 10
Gordon MacPherson *Bull Bugles*
Ian Mellish *Cairn*
John Godfrey *Demissus Spero*
Peter Garvey *Pedal*

The Clarion Band, John Godfrey (director)

Clive Wilkinson *Pollen Count* ☆☆☆
Michael Nyman *Time's Up*
Alec Roth *Full Fathom Five*
Peter Garvey *Sextet* ☆☆☆

Gamelan Setar Petak and aNeMonE

March 11
Vivienne Olive *Liebeslied*
Jonty Harrison *tremulous couplings*

Deborah Parker (vc), Henry Brown (pno)

March 12
Peter Seabourne *Plain Song* ☆☆☆
David Collins *Wanderers Nachtlied*
David Blake *Arias*
Stanley Hawkins *War Songs* ☆☆☆

Sandra Lissenden (sop), Andrew Sparling (cl),
and Katharine Durran (pno)

March 14
Philip Grange *La Ville Entière*
Corey Field *The Bright Shape of Sleep*
Judith Weir *Sketches from a Bagpiper's Album*

Alan Hacker (cl) and Karen Evans (pno)

William Sweeney *Trio*

Gordon MacPherson *Oh, why should I cry upon
my Wedding Day?* ☆☆☆; *The High Girders* ☆☆☆

Lesley Schatzberger (cl), Alan George (vla), Karen
Evans (pno), Elizabeth Haddon (vln), University
Orchestra, John Godfrey (director)

March 15
Electro-acoustic works

Jonty Stockdale *Inside-Out*
Ian Mellish *Hidden States*
Phil Ellis *Ritual*
Andrew Bentley *Aerial Views* ☆☆
Richard Orton *Astrorum Conscius* ☆☆☆
Tom Endrich *The Watcher's Orbit*
David Evan Jones *Scritto* ☆☆
Denis Smalley *Clarinet Threads* (with Roger
Heaton, cl)

March 16
Stephen Oliver *Ricercar*
Philip Wilby *And I move around the Cross*
David Blake *Cassation*
Tony Coe *Something Blue*
Mick Wilson *Dangerous Pleasure*

Royal Northern College of Music Wind Ensemble,
Timothy Reynish (director)

March 17
Roger Marsh *Music for Piano and Wind
Instruments* ☆☆☆

aNeMonE

March 18
David Collins *Quartet* ☆☆☆
John Paynter *Quartet*
Fitzwilliam String Quartet

March 19
Christopher Fox *auf dem Zweig*
Anthony Adams *9 Haikus*
Michael Parkin *Who is Anthea?*
Tom Endrich *Cartoon*

Soundpool

Derek Chivers *An English Clarinettist in
Venice* ☆☆☆

Alan Hacker (cl), York Area Schools Symphony
Orchestra, David Lloyd (director)

March 20
Harrison Birtwistle *Bow Down*

Northern Music Theatre

March 21
Wilfrid Mellers *Canticum Incarnationis*
Anthony Powers *Piano Sonata*

Vocal Ensemble, Peter Seymour (director), Paul
Roberts (pno)

Harrison Birtwistle *Melancolia I*
Michael Tippett *Symphony No. 2*

University Orchestra with Alan Hacker (cl), Graham
Treacher (director)

Park Lane Group – British String Quartet Series

Purcell Room

March 11
Priaulx Rainier *String Quartet*
Robert Walker *Quartet*
Robert Simpson *Quartet No. 2*

Delmé Quartet

March 18
George Nicholson *Quartet No. 2* ☆
Edward Cowie *Quartet No. 4 (Australia II)* ☆☆☆

Fairfield Quartet

March 25
Phyllis Tate *Movements for Quartet*
Timothy Murray *Quartet No. 1* ☆☆

Allegri Quartet

Bath Festival

Linley House, 1 Pierrepoint Place, Bath
Artistic Director: Amelia Freedman

May 25
Mark-Anthony Turnage *And still a softer morning*
Betsy Jolas *Quartet No. 2* ☆☆

Lontano, Sarah Leonard (sop), Odaline de la
Martinez (director)

May 27
Harrison Birtwistle *Secret Theatre*

Royal College of Music twentieth-century
ensemble, George Benjamin (director)

May 30
Paul Archbold *Aphrodite*
James Clarke *Downstream*
Mark-Anthony Turnage *Lament for a Hanging Man*
Javier Alvarez *Tientos*

Music Projects/London, Sarah Leonard (sop),
Richard Bernas (director)

June 3
Mark-Anthony Turnage *One Hand in Brooklyn
 Heights* (extracts) ☆☆☆

New London Chamber Choir, James Wood
(director)

June 6
Mark-Anthony Turnage *Entranced*

Ian Brown (pno)

June 7
Nicholas Maw *Personae* (complete version) ☆☆☆

Peter Donohoe (pno)

Aldeburgh Festival

Aldeburgh Foundation, Aldeburgh, Suffolk

June 7
Richard Rodney Bennett *Sonata*

Julian Bream (guitar)

June 9
Gordon Crosse *Wavesongs*

Alexander Baillie (vc), Ian Brown (pno)

June 10
Michael Tippett *Fantasia Concertante*

English Chamber Orchestra, Stuart Bedford
(director)

June 18
Rupert Bawden *Le Livre de Fauvel* ☆☆☆

London Sinfonietta, Oliver Knussen (director)

June 19
John Lambert *String Quartet*
Tributes to John Lambert from some of his pupil

London Sinfonietta, Oliver Knussen (director)

June 20
Colin Matthews *Suite for piano; Oboe Quartet*

Royal Northern College of Music students

June 21
Colin Matthews *Divertimento*

Britten-Pears Orchestra, Hugh Maguire (director)

St Magnus Festival

Orkney Islands
Artistic Director: Peter Maxwell Davies

June 20
Peter Maxwell Davies *The Lighthouse*

The Fires of London, Gunther Bauer-Schenk
(director)

June 21
Peter Maxwell Davies *Violin Concerto* ☆☆☆

Isaac Stern (vln), Royal Philharmonic Orchestra,
André Previn (director)

June 22
Peter Maxwell Davies *Jimmy the Postie* ☆☆☆

Royal Philharmonic Orchestra, Peter Maxwell
Davies (director)

June 23
Peter Maxwell Davies *The House of Winter* ☆☆☆

The Kings' Singers

Wilde Festival

South Hill Park Arts Centre, Bracknell, Berkshire
Artistic Director: Ron Macallister

June 28
Edward McGuire *String Trio* ☆☆☆

Nash Ensemble

June 29
Felix Ibarrondo *Brisas* ☆☆
Milton Babbitt *Head of the Bed* ☆☆
Joseph Schwantner *Sparrows* ☆☆

Lontano, with Jane Manning (sop), Odaline de la
Martinez (director)

Simon Bainbridge *Three Players*

Quorum
Ben Mason *Daughter of Fortune*
Sally Beamish *New work* ☆☆☆
Contraband
Milton Babbitt *String Quartet No. 3* ☆☆; *Don* ☆☆
Hanson String Quartet, Andrew Ball (pno)

Almeida Festival

Almeida Street, London N1
Artistic Director: Pierre Audi

The featured composers were Arvo Pärt and Steve Reich and there were celebrations of the music of Spain and Japan.

In addition to this rich repertoire there were the following British works:

June 20
James Dillon *Sgothan; Diffractions*

June 21
Brian Ferneyhough *Unity Capsule*

Pierre-Yves Artaud (fls)

June 22
New works for shakuhachi and electronics by Ian Dearden, Andrew Lewis, Michael Vaughan, and Michael Turnbull

Yoshikazu Iwamoto (shakuhachi)

Chris Dench *Topologies; Espérance; '. . . the caught breath of time'; Shunga* ☆☆☆; *Tilt*

Andrew Ball and Michael Finnissy (pnos), Nancy Ruffer (fl), Mary King (mezzo-sop), Simon Limbrick (perc), Christopher Redgate (ob)

June 23
Bach-Harrison Birtwistle *Five Chorale Preludes*
Oliver Knussen *Fragments from Chiara* ☆☆☆
Mark-Anthony Turnage *Lament for a Hanging Man*
Andrew Vores *New work* ☆☆☆
Peter Maxwell Davies *Agnus Dei* ☆☆☆

Almeida Festival Players, Oliver Knussen (director), BBC Singers, Simon Joly (director)

June 25
Jonathan Lloyd *Feuding Fiddles* ☆☆☆; *John's Journal; String Quartet* ☆☆☆; *It's All Sauce To Me; Mill of Memories; Almeida Dances* ☆☆☆

Almeida Festival Players with Yvar Mikhashoff and John Lenehan (pnos) and John Harle (sax)

James Wood *Barong* ☆

Andrew Ball, Julian Jacobson (pnos), Simon Limbrick and James Wood (perc)

June 27
Oliver Knussen *Music for The Saxon Shore* ☆☆☆
Geoffrey King *Sonata for two pianos* ☆

Almeida Festival Players, Oliver Knussen (director)

John White *12 Sonatas* ☆☆☆
Ben Mason *New Work* ☆☆☆
Dave Smith *Recuerdos* ☆☆☆

John White (pno)

June 29
Michael Nyman *Zoo Caprices* ☆☆☆

Alexander Balanescu (vln)

June 30
James Wood *Ho shang Yao; Usas* ☆☆☆; *Choroi kai Thaliai*

July 2
James Wood *String Quartet; T'ien chung Yao*

July 6
James Wood *Phaedrus* ☆☆☆

Electric Phoenix, Sara Stowe (sop), James Wood, Simon Limbrick, and Robyn Schulkowsky (perc), David Wilson-Johnson (bar), New London Chamber Choir, New London Percussion Ensemble, Endymion Ensemble, Arditti Quartet, John Whiting (electronics), James Wood (director)

Cheltenham Festival

Town Hall, Cheltenham, Gloucestershire
Artistic Director: John Manduell

July 5
Alun Hoddinott *Triple Concerto* ☆☆☆

Stuttgart Piano Trio, BBC Philharmonic Orchestra, Alun Hoddinott (director)

July 9
Robert Saxton *Viola Concerto* ☆☆☆

Paul Silverthorne (vla), Scottish Chamber Orchestra, Wilfried Boettcher (director)

July 12
William Kraft *Weavings* ☆☆

Kronos Quartet with Peter Sadlo (perc)

July 13
Peter Racine Fricker *A Wish for a Party*
Lennox Berkeley *Three Songs for Four Male Voices*
Alun Hoddinott *Hymnus ante somnum*

The Schubertians, Carl Zytowski (director)

July 14
Lennox Berkeley *String Trio*

Goldberg Ensemble

July 15
Peter Racine Fricker *Five Studies*

Neil Rutman (pno)

Michael Berkeley *Songs of Awakening Love* ☆☆☆

Heather Harper (sop), City of London Sinfonia, Richard Hickox (director)

July 17
Richard Rodney Bennett *Duo Concertant* ☆☆☆

Nicholas Cox (cl), Vanessa Latarche (pno)

July 18
William Kraft *Interplay* ☆☆

City of Birmingham Symphony Orchestra, Simon Rattle (director)

July 20
Peter Racine Fricker *Concerto for orchestra* ☆☆☆

Royal Philharmonic Orchestra, Antal Dorati (director)

Kings Lynn Festival
The Fermoy Centre, King Street, Kings Lynn, Norfolk

July 26
Tristan Murail *New work for synthesiser and computer* ☆☆☆
Jonathan Harvey *Mortuos Plango, Vivos Voco*
George Benjamin *Panorama*

Tristan Murail and Francoise Pellie-Murail (synthesisers and computer)

July 27
Oliver Knussen *Ophelia Dances*
Tristan Murail *Territoires de l'oubli* ☆☆
George Benjamin *At First Light*

Downshire Players, Peter Ash (director)

July 29
George Benjamin *Three Studies for piano*
Pierre Boulez *Memorial . . . Explosante-fixe* ☆☆

George Benjamin (pno), Divertimenti, George Benjamin (director)

July 30
George Benjamin *Altitude*

Grimethorpe Colliery Band, David James (director)

July 31
George Benjamin *A Mind of Winter*

Teresa Cahill (sop), Northern Sinfonia, George Benjamin (director)

London Sinfonietta/Summerscope Festival
Queen Elizabeth Hall
Artistic Director: Michael Vyner

August 8
Dominic Muldowney *Sinfonietta* ☆☆☆
Steve Martland *Orc*
Mark-Anthony Turnage *On All Fours*
Simon Holt *. . . era madrugada*
George Benjamin *At First Light*

Frank Lloyd (hn), John Harle (saxs), Christopher van Kampen (vc), Diego Masson (director)

Edinburgh Festival
A weekend of twentieth-century music devised by Alexander Goehr

August 22
Peter Maxwell Davies *String Quartet No. 1*
Harrison Birtwistle *Clarinet Quintet*
Alexander Goehr *String Quartet No. 3*

Nicholas Cox (cl), Brodsky String Quartet

August 23
Alexander Goehr *Sonata about Jerusalem*

Scottish Chamber Orchestra, Richard Bernas (director)

Philip Cashian *Moon of the Dawn* ☆☆☆

Carol Smith (sop), Brodsky String Quartet

August 24
Charles Wuorinen *Capriccio* ☆☆
Roger Sessions *Piano Sonata No. 3* ☆☆

Alan Feinberg (pno)

August 25
Hugh Wood *Quintet*
Bayan Northcott *Sextet*
Anthony Gilbert *Quartet of Beasts*
Geoffrey King *You, Always You* ☆☆☆
Nicholas Sackman *Corranach*

Lontano, Odaline de la Martinez (director)

Concert Series, 1985–6
New Macnaghten Concerts
64 Highgate High Street, London N6
Chairman: Andrew Morris

October 1   St John's, Smith Square
Steve Martland *Orc* ☆☆
Gary Carpenter *Die Flimmerkiste*

Lontano with Stefan Blonk (hn), Odaline de la Martinez (director)

October 29   St John's, Smith Square
Gavin Bryars *My First Hommage*
John White *The Oppo Contained*
Dave Smith *A Gay Romp*
Ben Mason, Dave Smith, and John White *Garden Furniture Music*

December 3   St John's, Smith Square
Bill Hopkins Tribute Concert

Bill Hopkins *Two Pomes; Sensation; Pendant*
Roger Redgate *. . . of torn pathways . . .* ☆☆☆

January 21   The Place Theatre
Turning Point Ensemble
Performance Art

March 11   The Place Theatre
The Orchestra of Lights with Evan Parker (sax)
Improvisation

The Americas
Series of concerts given by Lontano, directed by Odaline de la Martinez at St John's, Smith Square

October 15
Paul Lansky *As If* ☆☆
Judith Weir *The Consolations of Scholarship* ☆
Roger Reynolds *Transfigured Wind III* ☆☆

November 25
John Hopkins *White Winter, Black Spring* ☆
Serge Garant *Quintette* ☆☆
Bernard Rands *Canti del Sole* ☆

December 19
Silvestre Revueltas *First and Second Little Serious Pieces* ☆☆
Marisa Rezende *Sexteto em seis Tempos* ☆☆
Charles Wuorinen *Speculum Speculi* ☆☆
Odaline de la Martinez *Cantos de amor* ☆

January 23
Guillermo Rendon *Serkan Ikala* ☆☆
Leon Biriotti *Concierto para Oboe* ☆☆
Peter Lieberson *Lalita* ☆☆
Nicholas Sackman *Corronach* ☆☆☆

Scottish Chamber Orchestra 'Composer Conducts' Series
Queen's Hall, Edinburgh

November 14
Harrison Birtwistle *Songs by Myself; Carmen Arcadiae Mechanicae Perpetuum*

December 7
Oliver Knussen *Music for a Puppet Court; Second Symphony*

February 26
Peter Maxwell Davies *Sinfonia*

March 22
Edward Harper *Fantasia EH3 7DC; Intrada after Monteverdi*

April 10
Peter Maxwell Davies *Into the Labyrinth*

Music of Eight Decades
October 30   Queen Elizabeth Hall
Colin Matthews *Suns Dance* ☆☆☆
Charles Wuorinen *Canzona* ☆☆
Peter Maxwell Davies *Revelation and Fall*

London Sinfonietta with Linda Hirst (mezzo-sop), Oliver Knussen (director)

December 3   Royal Festival Hall
York Höller *Piano Concerto* ☆☆☆
Bernard Rands *Le Tambourin* ☆☆

BBC Symphony Orchestra with Peter Donohoe (pno), Elgar Howarth and Bernard Rands (directors)

December 11   Royal Festival Hall
George Benjamin *Ringed by the Flat Horizon*
David Matthews *In the Dark Time* ☆☆☆

BBC Symphony Orchestra, Mark Elder (director)

January 29   Royal Festival Hall
Toru Takemitsu *riverrun* ☆☆

BBC Symphony Orchestra, David Atherton (director)

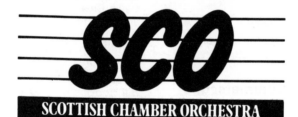

March 5   Queen Elizabeth Hall
Tristan Murail *Les Courants de l'Espace* ☆☆
Robert Saxton *Chamber Symphony: Circles of Light* ☆☆☆

London Sinfonietta, Esa-Pekka Salonen (director)

March 14   Royal Festival Hall
Bernd Alois Zimmerman *Dialoge* ☆☆
Harrison Birtwistle *Earth Dances* ☆☆☆

BBC Symphony Orchestra with Bruno Canino and Antonio Ballista (pnos), Peter Eötvös (director)

April 2   Queen Elizabeth Hall
Witold Lutoslawski *Chain 2* ☆☆
Brian Ferneyhough *Carceri d'Invenzione I*

London Sinfonietta with Gyorgy Pauk (vln), Diego Masson and Witold Lutoslawski (directors)

June 4   Queen Elizabeth Hall
James Dillon *Uberschreiten* ☆☆☆

London Sinfonietta, Lothar Zagrosek (director)

Four Composers – Endymion Ensemble Series
Purcell Room

December 19
Oliver Knussen *Masks; Three Little Fantasies; Océan de terre; Hums and Songs of Winnie-the-Pooh; Autumnal; Ophelia Dances*
Oliver Knussen and John Whitfield (directors)

January 23
Simon Bainbridge *People of the Dawn; Music for Mel and Nora; Voicing; Three Pieces for chamber ensembles; Concertante in moto perpetuo; Three Players* ☆☆☆
Simon Bainbridge and John Whitfield (directors)

February 20
Dominic Muldowney *Five Theatre Poems; A Second Show; The Duration of Exile; Chorale Preludes* ☆☆☆
Dominic Muldowney and John Whitfield (directors)

March 20
Nigel Osborne *I am Goya; Mythologies; Alba; Remembering Esenin; Piano Sonata; Zansa*
Nigel Osborne and John Whitfield (directors)

Úroboros Ensemble
55 Belmont Road, St Andrew's, Bristol
Artistic Director: Gwyn Pritchard
St John's, Smith Square

February 19
Toshi Ichiyanagi *Recurrence* ☆☆
Michael Finnissy *Câtana* ☆
Gwyn Pritchard *Moondance* ☆

March 19
David Bedford *Pentaquin* ☆
Edwin Roxburgh *Dithyramb* ☆

Helmut Lachenmann *Trio Fluido* ☆☆
Peter Nelson *Quartet for flute, clarinet, viola, and harp* ☆

April 16
Gwyn Pritchard *Chamber Concerto* ☆
Michael Travlos *Progressions for solo oboe* ☆☆
Alfred Nieman *Soliloquy for solo cello* ☆☆☆
Robert Saxton *The Sentinel of the Rainbow*

Arts Council Contemporary Music Network
105 Piccadilly, London W1
Co-ordinator: Annette Morreau
(Programmes toured around the UK)

The Vienna Art Orchestra
   The Minimalism of Erik Satie
Electronic Music Now
   Nigel Osborne *New work for mezzo-sop and tape*
   Denis Smalley *Tides*
   Marco Stroppa *Traiettoria*
   Jean-Claude Risset *Inharmonique*
   Tim Souster *Work for computer-operating pianist*

   Linda Hirst (mezzo-sop), Denis Smalley (sound projection), Philip Mead (pno), Tim Souster (director and electronics)

Anthony Braxton Quartet
Orchestra of St John's, Smith Square
   Arnold Schoenberg *Chamber Symphony No. 2*
   Peter Maxwell Davies *Sinfonia Concertante*
   Alfred Schnittke *Violin Concerto No. 2*
   Brahms *Serenade No. 2*

   Mark Lubotsky (vln), John Lubbock (director)

Capricorn
   Alfred Schnittke *Piano Quintet*
   David Blake *Clarinet Quintet*
   György Ligeti *Horn Trio*

Steve Reich and Musicians
   Steve Reich *Vermont Counterpoint; Clapping Music; Drumming Part III; New York Counterpoint* ☆☆; *Sextet* ☆☆

London Sinfonietta
   Toru Takemitsu *Rain Coming*
   Harrison Birtwistle *Secret Theatre*
   Kurt Weill *Suite from the Threepenny Opera*
   Toru Takemitsu *Rain Spell*

   Diego Masson (director)

Tony Oxley/Didier Levallet
   Anglo-French Double Quartet

MusICA
ICA, The Mall, London SW1
Artistic Director: Adrian Jack

July 6
Helmut Lachenmann *Salut für Caudwell; Mouvement for ensemble*

119

Circle, Ingo Metzmacher (director), Wilhelm Bruck and Theodor Ross (guitars)

July 13
Wolfgang Rihm *String Quartet No. 7*
LaMonte Young *Five Small Pieces*
Mel Graves *Pangaea*
Jin Hi Kim *Linkings*
Kevin Volans *White Man Sleeps*

Kronos Quartet

July 20
Javier Alvarez *Redobles* ☆☆☆
Jesús Alvarez *Sarabanda* ☆☆☆
David Sawer *Cat's Eye* ☆☆☆

Lontano, Odaline de la Martinez (director)

September 7
György Ligeti *Horn Trio; Études*
László Vidovsky *Horn Trio*

Alan Feinberg (pno), Rolf Schulte (vln), William Purvis (hn)

Lontano 10th Anniversary Concerts
Queen Elizabeth Hall

May 14
Steve Martland *American Invention* ☆
Richard Rodney Bennett *Jazz Calendar*

June 2
Steve Martland *Remembering Lennon* (revised version) ☆

Lontano, Odaline de la Martinez (director)

Henry Wood Promenade Concerts
Artistic Director: John Drummond (BBC Controller, Music)
Royal Albert Hall

July 25
Hans Werner Henze *Symphony No. 7* ☆☆

City of Birmingham Symphony Orchestra, Simon Rattle (director)

July 28
Alun Hoddinott *The sun, the great luminary of the universe*

BBC Welsh Symphony Orchestra, Alun Hoddinott (director)

July 29
Michael Tippett *Concerto for Orchestra*

London Sinfonietta, Andrew Davis (director)

August 1
George Benjamin *A Mind of Winter*

Teresa Cahill (sop), Northern Sinfonia, George Benjamin (director)

John Casken *To fields we do not know*
Giles Swayne *Missa Tiburtina* (complete) ☆☆☆

BBC Singers, John Poole (director)

August 4
Nigel Osborne *The Sickle*

Jane Manning (sop), City of London Sinfonia, Richard Hickox (director)

August 9
Gordon Crosse *Array for trumpet and strings*

Håkan Hardenberger (tpt), BBC Welsh Symphony Orchestra, James Loughran (director)

August 15
Oliver Knussen *Fragments from Chiara*
Alexander Goehr *a musical offering (J.S.B. 1985)*

BBC Singers, Simon Joly (director), London Sinfonietta, Oliver Knussen (director)

August 20
Peter Dickinson *Piano Concerto*

Howard Shelley (pno), BBC Symphony Orchestra, David Atherton (director)

August 23
Nicholas Maw *Sonata for strings and horns*

London Mozart Players, Jane Glover (director)

August 27
Jonathan Harvey *Madonna of Winter and Spring* ☆☆☆
Harrison Birtwistle *Earth Dances*

BBC Symphony Orchestra, Peter Eötvös (director)

September 3
John Casken *Orion Over Farne* ☆

Scottish National Orchestra, Matthias Bamert (director)

September 6
John Maxwell Geddes *Voyager*

BBC Scottish Symphony Orchestra, Jerzy Maksymiuk (director)